Prevention

EASY
Resistance
Band
SLIM-DOWN

Prevention

EASY
Resistance
Band
SLIM-DOWN

The low-impact way to get leaner and stronger in 28 days

Kymberly Nolden, C.P.T. and the editors of Prevention

Contents

Introduction

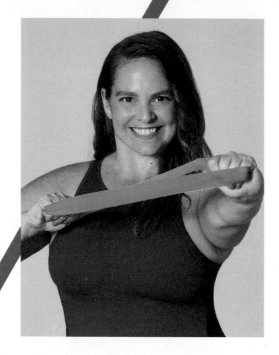

Hi!

My name is Kymberly and ever since I can remember, I've loved movement. To this day, a favorite part of my job as a personal trainer is watching someone figure out how to do an exercise and discovering how that affects them beyond the feat they just achieved. Simply put, good movement helps you feel good. I'm fascinated by all the ways the human body can move, and by finding ways to help all bodies move better.

I'm a trauma-informed personal trainer and mobility specialist, and my journey began when I got my B.A. in dance and movement analysis. (Is there any greater joy than just shaking it to a great song?) I later went on to become the fitness facility manager at Einstein Medical College, where my main job is developing our group fitness, personal training, and coaching programs.

As I was creating workouts for all kinds of people, I encountered a not-so-fun reality. We all, at one point or another, face an obstacle that threatens to make physical activity difficult. I've worked with clients dealing with acute pain, clients with chronic pain, and, most commonly, clients whose busy lives leave them feeling stressed at the thought of squeezing in daily movement.

Sound familiar? We've all had that feeling of being overwhelmed. We've all felt daunted by the task of fitting everything in when our lives are already packed to the brim. Maybe you don't always have one large block of time to work out. Or maybe you have the time, but chronic pain leaves you worried that lifting weights or getting on the treadmill will make things worse. Often I see clients stuck in a cycle of adopting extreme and unsustainable exercise and diet plans. When life throws them a curveball, they abandon the plan, feel guilty, and then try to recommit. Eventually every Monday becomes more restricted, and every weekend feels more uncontrollable.

This cycle, the sense that you've failed, and unrealistic expectations—followed by guilt for not having the willpower to see those goals through—often leads straight to burnout. Also it can bring you to the absolutely false belief that you're lazy. This is not a mindset that's conducive to success in anything. Yet, it's a cycle that so many of us have fallen into.

There is a way to break that cycle—to make a commitment to yourself that is not only doable, but makes you feel great. I created a 28-day plan that I hope will help you see the changes you want in not only your body, but also your mind. To help you celebrate every little action you do for your health while not sweating missing a workout or struggling with an exercise.

To do that, you'll be working with what I consider to be one of the most fun fitness tools out there: the resistance band. These bands are inexpensive, portable, joint-friendly, and great for safely building total-body strength. I'll show you how to use them to lose weight, prevent pain, and improve your range of motion so you feel better moving in everyday life. Plus, I'll show you how to do it all in just 18 minutes.

You're also going to learn how to approach fitness with a more flexible attitude so you can ease up on the pressure and just have fun. As you'll see in Chapter 3, you can customize this plan to your schedule and physical ability. After all, you could have the most well-thought-out workout plan, but if it's not adaptable—especially when life throws you a curveball—you won't see the results you want or results you can maintain.

So instead, I say let's start having fun first and foremost! The rest will follow, I promise.

Kymberly Nolden, C.P.T.

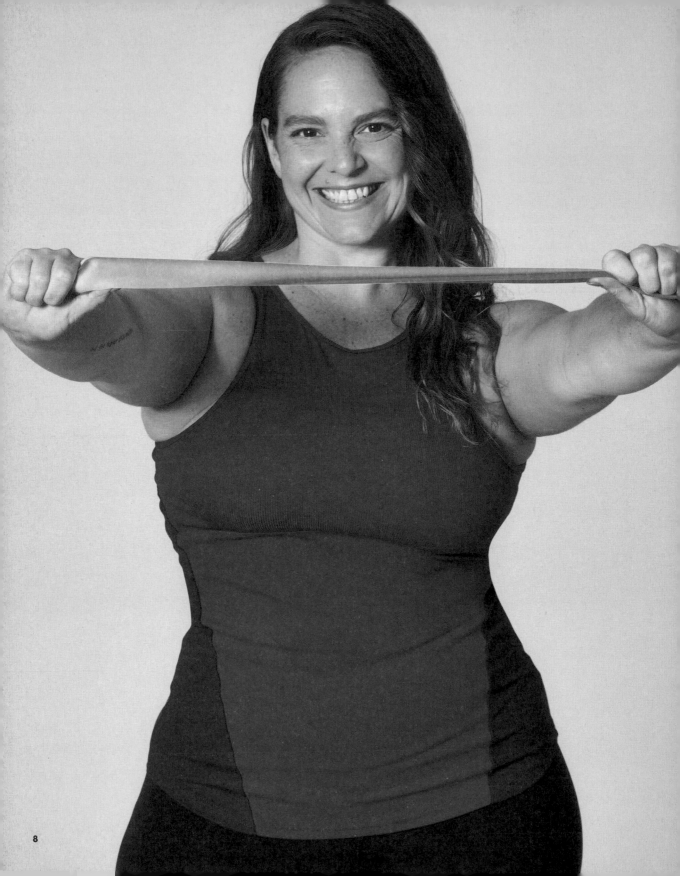

01

The Power of Resistance Bands

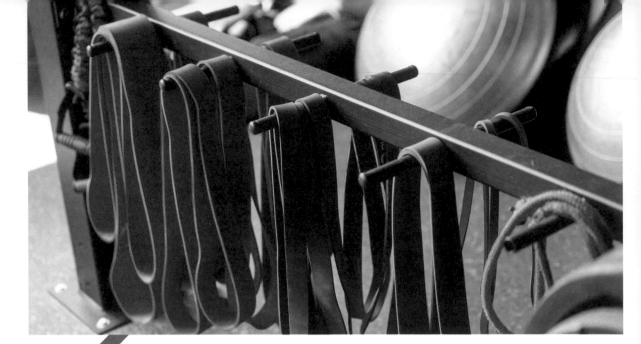

When it comes to working out and achieving noticeable results, it's all too easy to buy into the old adage "Go big or go home." Lift heavy dumbbells, hop on that expensive stationary bike, or sweat it out on a bulky weight machine at the gym. But here's the truth: You don't need all that stuff to get strong, burn fat, and improve your mobility.

All you need is a tool that's small enough to fit in your purse: a resistance band. Made from thin, ultra-stretchy material such as rubber or latex, resistance bands typically weigh less than a pound but can generate resistance dozens of times their own weight. They're typically flat or tubular and come in a wide variety of types to suit your exercise routine and fitness level. For example, some bands are open-ended, allowing you to tie one side to an anchor when you do pulling exercises. Others come in the form of a loop so you can securely add resistance to exercises like donkey kicks. They come in various levels of resistance, and their essential function is to create an opposing force on your muscles, which in turn helps you build strength.

For the program in this book, you'll want a set of mini loop bands, long loop bands, and long, open-ended bands. For the mini loop bands, I suggest purchasing both rubber and fabric types. That's because rubber bands, which are great for around the arches of your feet or wrists, tend to roll when used around your legs or upper arms. Fabric bands, for their part, tend to feel bulky on your feet and wrists. But they don't roll, so they feel more comfortable and secure during exercises involving your legs and upper arms.

Aside from being lightweight, compact, and affordable, resistance bands are incredibly versatile and can be used for almost any exercise in the place of other forms of weight or resistance. For a long time, bands were found mostly in physical therapy facilities and used for rehab exercises due to their value in gently rebuilding awareness of your surroundings. (More on that later.) Today, however, they're used outside of PT clinics for all sorts of exercises to improve everything from strength to mobility.

Why You'll Love Resistance Bands

This lightweight tool is a heavy hitter when it comes to boosting fitness. Here are a few reasons why I love using them—and why you will too!

THEY'RE LIKE HAVING 10 WEIGHTS IN ONE

Strength training is essential to maintaining your health as you get older, but buying and storing a full set of weights isn't always feasible—or affordable. With a resistance band, you can mimic the effects of using a whole range of dumbbells just by adjusting your grip or the placement of the band. Say you're doing a pull-apart (which you'll learn on page 85), and after a few reps you notice that keeping proper form is becoming more difficult. If you were using dumbbells, you might need to drop them and switch to a lighter pair. Using a band, you can simply move your hands farther apart to decrease the resistance and continue to your goal rep range without sacrificing form. This makes bands ideal for anyone who isn't sure what level of resistance to start with on their strength-training journey. No need to invest in a pile of weights that might not be the right fit! I especially like using resistance bands with clients who need to improve their joint health, especially older individuals, post-injury clients, and women who are pregnant or recently gave birth. If you fall into one of these groups, you may feel like some days your workouts are easy, and some days they're not. Just like bands can make an exercise easier, they can also make a move more challenging. For example, you

can wrap a long band around your upper back as you do push-ups to add resistance to the movement. With bands, adjusting the difficulty of your workout is super simple, even in the middle of an exercise!

THEY MAKE IT EASY TO GET YOUR FORM RIGHT

Ever get halfway through a workout and wonder, "Am I even doing this right?" Proper form, or the way you position your body as you go through the motions of an exercise, is crucial to getting the maximum benefit and limiting your risk of injury. A band can remind your body of form cues so you perform a movement better and without pain, which means you're strengthening your joints and muscles more efficiently and safely. For example, you might loop a mini band around your arms to prevent your elbows from flaring out during a pushup. Think of these bands like bumpers on a bowling lane guiding your ball.

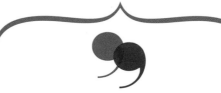

With a resistance band, you can mimic the effects of using a whole range of dumbbells just by adjusting your grip or the placement of the band.

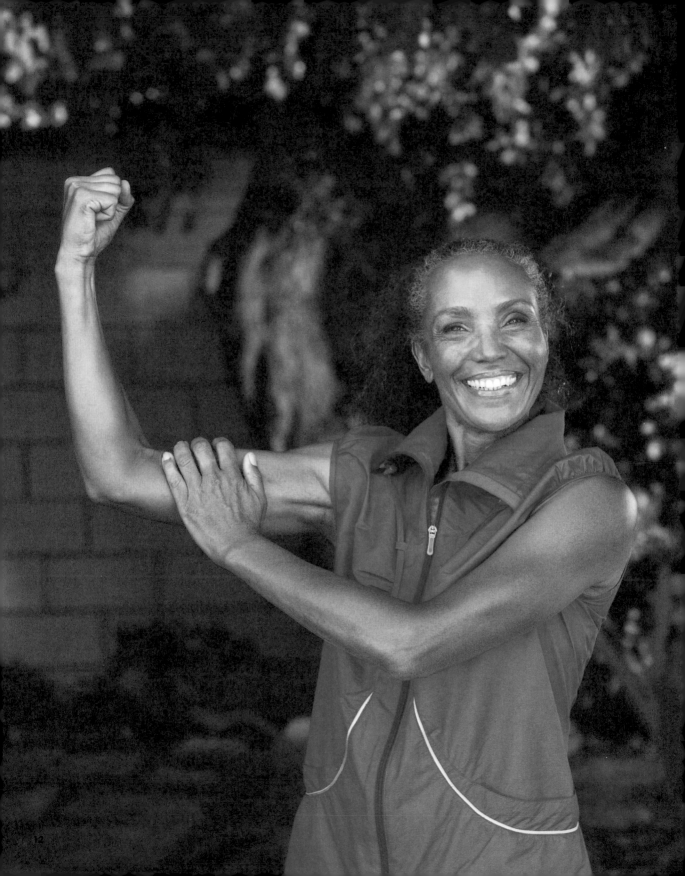

THEY'RE GENTLE ON YOUR JOINTS

Speaking of joint health, bands are fantastic tools for anyone who wants to prevent or limit joint pain while working out. Your joints get stronger just like your muscles do. Due to the bands' stretchy nature, your body needs to work harder to stabilize, as well as go through the entire range of motion, than if you were using rigid weights. This bonus is one reason why bands are especially helpful for your joints— building joint strength requires stabilizing exercises. Bands can also help ease joint stress during high-impact movements. Once a client progresses from an injury or gains enough strength, I like to add bands to body weight exercises to help them mimic the effects of plyometric (explosive) movement, such as jumps, but without any of the actual jumping! This helps them master their technique and alleviates potential joint strain.

THEY HELP YOU BUILD AND MAINTAIN MUSCLE

The resistance band exercises in the 28-day program can help you grow muscle and get stronger without ever hoisting anything heavy overhead. That's especially important for older people, because we begin to naturally lose muscle mass with age. Building and preserving muscle not only supports weight management (which we'll discuss in the next section), but also assists a whole range of other vital functions. For example, as you get older, adequate muscle mass can help protect your mobility (that is, how easily you move through daily life), reducing your odds of injuring yourself during everyday tasks.

Muscle can also affect everything from how well you recover from movement to your mental and emotional health and even your cognitive functioning. In fact, protecting your muscles can literally help prevent cognitive decline, as a 2023 study in the journal *GeroScience* suggests. Researchers who had 60- to 80-year-olds perform resistance exercises twice a week for 12 weeks noted that by the study's end, the area of the participants' brains that helps preserve cognitive health had been positively altered. Talk about getting strong head to toe!

THEY LOWER YOUR RISK OF INJURY

Nothing can completely prevent injury—accidents can happen. However, you can cheat the odds. How? By building strong muscles and joints, you'll improve your ability to react to your surroundings. Resistance bands are especially helpful in training kinesthetic awareness and proprioception— that is, your sense of generally where your body is in the space around you. That's because no matter which way you move with a band, you're encountering an opposing force, bringing your attention to your body. In other words, it's pretty hard to simply go through the motions while doing these exercises. Developing these skills can help you respond more quickly when, say, you encounter a bump in the sidewalk. You're more likely to catch yourself if you trip or even avoid stumbling altogether. Bands also offer a safe and gentle way to take your workouts to the next level. To progress in your fitness journey, you can't keep lifting the same load over and over again. But sometimes

> ### DID YOU KNOW?
> When compared to dumbbells, resistance bands have been shown to work some muscles even more than weights! A 2018 study in *The Journal of Human Kinetics* found that when participants performed flys and delt flys with bands they activated some shoulder and back muscles more than when they performed the same moves with dumbbells.

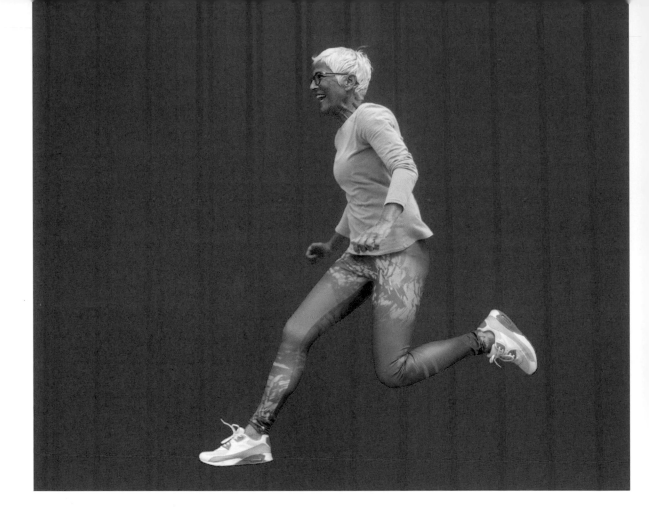

the next step can feel like a giant leap from your current abilities, leaving you vulnerable to injury. Bands ease the transition. Remember my tip about adjusting your grip on the band? That's one way to customize any move to your comfort level.

THEY KEEP YOUR WORKOUTS FUN

Fact: There are only so many squats you can do before you get bored. Add a resistance band and suddenly you have a half dozen new ways to perform the same tried-and-true move (and new opportunities to hit your muscles from different angles). It's all about varying your lines of pull, or the direction from which you're pulling a resisting force. When you work out with a weight, like a dumbbell or kettlebell, you're limited to one line of pull:

vertical. That's because gravity will always pull the weight straight down. To lift the weight, you'll always have to pull straight up. Other resistance training tools, such as a cable machine or a landmine, can offer more lines of pull but still anchor you to the machine. Resistance bands, on the other hand, are nearly limitless. They don't have to be anchored to anything, and their line of pull will be dependent upon the exercise and placement. This means you could perform the same exercise but change the load countless ways simply by using different bands or placing the band in different positions. To shake up your squats, for instance, you could slip a loop slightly above your knees or stand on an open band while holding the ends at your shoulders. If you're someone who struggles with boredom doing the exact same exercise every week, bands allow you to play with different variations so you can continue to improve your squat while keeping your mind engaged as well. Which, even for us trainers, is essential to staying motivated and consistent!

Resistance Bands and Weight Loss

Because of their approachability, versatility, and ability to promote muscle growth, resistance bands can be a great tool for anyone looking to shed pounds and keep them off. To achieve safe, sustainable weight loss, it's important to understand what actually happens when you lose weight and what role your workout plays. When you know more about the process, it can mean the difference between falling into a pattern of yo-yo weight fluctuations and finally finding long-term success. Luckily, as long as you focus on giving your body what it needs, you can perform a rebalancing act, in a sense, with your muscle-to-fat ratio. Below, I'll explain how we do that in this program.

HOW YOUR BODY BURNS CALORIES

First, let's debunk a common myth about weight loss. Chances are you've heard someone say something along the lines of "If you eat one Oreo, you'll have to do 100 jumping jacks to burn it off." That's not exactly how the equation works. It's true that if you take in more calories than you burn, you'll store the excess as fat. And if you burn more calories than you take in, you'll use your stored fat to make up the difference in energy needed versus energy consumed. This leads to weight loss.

What makes this equation more complex, however, is that burning calories involves more than just jumping jacks and burpees. Your body uses energy in many other ways too, such as through your basal metabolic rate (BMR), non-exercise activity thermogenesis (NEAT),

exercise activity thermogenesis (EAT), digestion, and finally sleep and recovery. Your BMR is the energy needed to power every chemical reaction that happens in your body (essentially, the calories you burn just by existing). NEAT includes all the little ways you move every day that aren't part of your workouts, such as washing dishes or grocery shopping. EAT, on the other hand, includes what you may traditionally think of as exercise—running, swimming, lifting weights, and the very resistance band moves in this plan. What this all means is that you don't

With this plan, you can meet your goals without sacrificing all your time to exercise.

have to live at the gym to lose weight. Calorie burn takes many different forms. Which is why we've built the 28-day plan with a mix of NEAT and EAT so you can meet your goals without sacrificing all your time to exercise. Quick fun fact for you: Most of the body fat you lose when you lose weight doesn't leave through the bathroom or your sweat. As your stored fat gets broken down to be used, a small part of it breaks down into water (which is either absorbed or leaves your body through sweat and pee); the rest of it becomes carbon dioxide (CO_2) and leaves your body as you exhale.

MUSCLE'S MANY BENEFITS

So what does this all have to do with the resistance band workout plan you've decided to try? The exercises you'll be doing are especially good for building muscle. And building muscle, in turn, can boost your BMR, or the calories you burn when you're not engaging in physical activity. Muscle uses more energy than fat mass just to function, which means that even now, as you're reading this, your muscles are burning calories. Talk about more bang for your buck! But that doesn't mean you should focus exclusively on resistance training. Cardio is a crucial part of any well-rounded fitness routine. It boosts heart health, improves blood flow, and is just plain fun! You'll get your cardio in during this plan through activities like walking, hiking, or swimming—it's up to you! Coupled with the power of building muscle, you'll be on the road to safe and sustainable weight loss in no time.

 Of course, weight loss isn't the only reason you should think about building muscle. Muscle does so much more for your overall health! Shifting your focus to those benefits— instead of, say, the number on the scale—can keep you motivated on your toughest days so you stick with your fitness routine long-term. For example, if one of your life goals is to keep up with little ones, muscle can get you there. Muscle makes it easier to give piggyback rides and quickly get off the ground during a game of Duck, Duck, Goose. Your core muscles support your balance, reducing your risk of falls. Resistance training can even increase bone density, lowering your odds of developing osteoporosis. It all adds up to being able to live your life more fully—which is a more fun goal to strive for anyway.

The Truth About Resistance Training

Even with all these benefits, I often get pushback from folks who come to me for weight loss when they hear me talk about building muscle. That's simply because there's a lot of confusion out there about what building muscle means. For many, the image of a bodybuilder—bulging biceps, chiseled quads—comes to mind. While that kind of physique does come from resistance training, achieving it requires significantly more time, resistance, and effort than the plan you'll follow in this guidebook. You would have to not only work out for long sessions multiple times a week, but also strategically cycle your nutrition plan between eating a caloric surplus and

BURN MORE WITHOUT BURNING OUT	BMR	EAT	NEAT	CARDIO
You can lose weight without working out every day. My plan taps into four smarter ways to use energy:	Boost the calories you burn powering your body's vital functions (a.k.a. BMR) by building muscle. This plan helps you do it without ever lifting a weight.	Any weight-loss plan needs EAT, the calories you burn from exercise. I'll show you easy moves to make every workout fun.	Movement not categorized as exercise, NEAT helps you burn calories doing everyday activities. I've built in reminders to help you move more daily.	Regular cardio supports your heart and your weight-loss goals. On this plan you'll go beyond the treadmill with activities like hiking and cycling.

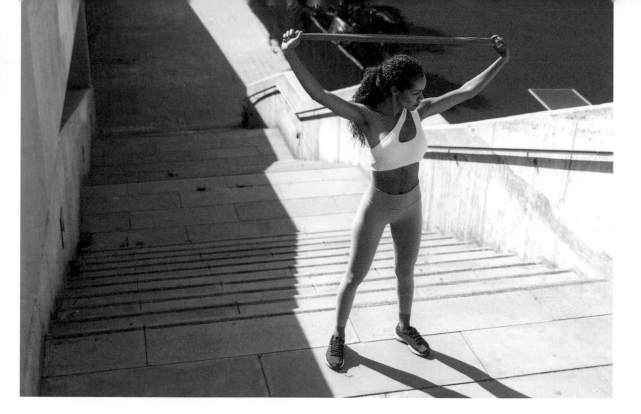

rather intense bouts of caloric deficits. Plus, the process takes years. On average, the maximum muscle mass a person can gain is two pounds a month—and that's on the high end, mostly seen in men and AMAB (assigned male at birth) persons, as well as those who are new to resistance training or who've taken a break from it. For everyone else, that average monthly gain is more like a half pound to a pound. On this plan, you'll build strength and moderate amounts of muscle, depending on where you're starting. And when you add muscle, you'll use more energy throughout the day, which means you've tipped that scale in favor of weight loss. Your clothes will fit better and your overall fitness will improve.

Many people say their goal is to get "toned" instead of building muscle. But here's the big secret: Getting toned and gaining muscle are the *same* thing. It's just that one phrase tends to conjure up images of bulky biceps, while the other suggests a more subtle muscle definition. In fact, muscle has only two options: It can get stronger and bigger, or it can atrophy and become weaker. Whether you call it building muscle or getting toned, you're

ultimately gaining muscle and strength—and that's a good thing! Also, the idea isn't just to build muscle beneath your stored body fat, but to use that muscle to then burn more calories at rest, using stored fat. So yes, you do grow muscle, but with this plan, you're also letting go of what you no longer need—body fat.

So to recap: Resistance bands are an incredible tool for building muscle, and muscle can help you lose weight—but most importantly, muscle boosts your overall health (from balance to bone density). That's why this plan focuses so much on just showing up. If you focus only on the "side effects" of your efforts (like losing weight) instead of how movement can improve your daily life (and make you feel good!), you run the risk of abandoning your new lifestyle once you hit your first life curveball. And that's not the way to achieve sustainable, long-term weight management. Focus on doing what makes your body stronger. Your weight will adjust eventually, as you continue to give your body what it needs in order to do what you ask of it. **In short: Trust the process!**

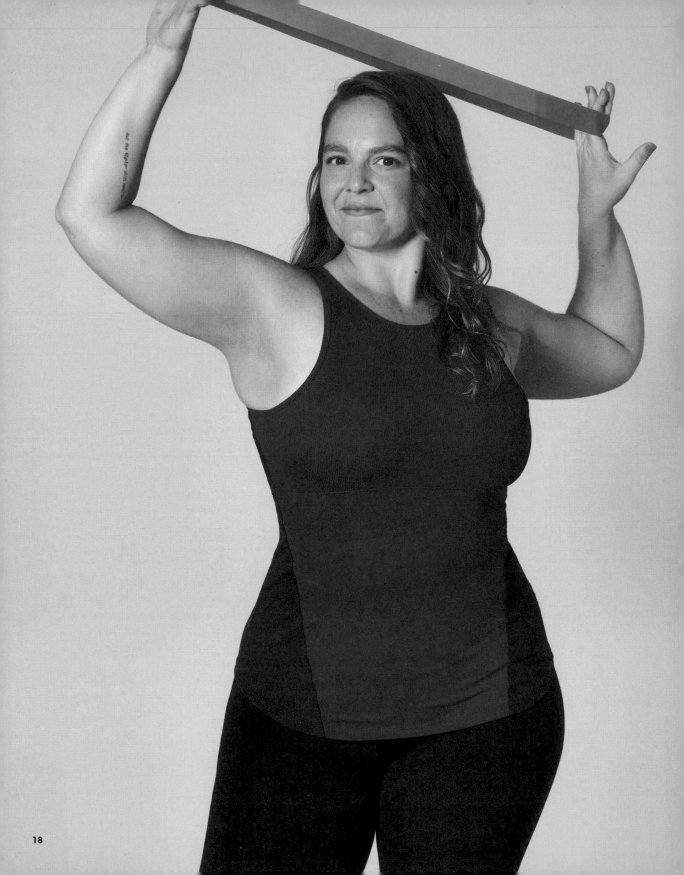

02

How to Get Real Results

We've all been there: It's Day 12 of a new health regimen that up to this point felt totally doable but now seems about as appealing as a trip to the DMV. Maintaining the motivation you need to see real results can be hard. The trick is incorporating little strategies to boost your physical and mental energy so you'll feel excited, or at least able, to complete each day of the plan. It's unrealistic to think that you'll always want to put in the work, even if you enjoy the work. That's why this plan is designed with flexibility in mind—to help you stay consistent when it feels tough to start, but also to allow you to push yourself or try new things when you have the energy to do so.

The tips I've outlined here will not only keep your spirits high (or serve as an anchor to remind yourself of the future reward of even doing the minimum) but also amp up your results during this program. My core piece of advice for reaching any fitness goal? Prioritize fulfilling your body's needs first. Help your body and mind function at their fullest potential throughout the next 28 days by following these guidelines.

MEASURE YOURSELF (BUT NOT THE WAY YOU THINK)

First, let's talk about mindset. Before you even do your very first rep, your mind has likely already been hard at work, contemplating everything from how difficult the workout might be to how many pounds you'll lose. Instead of meticulously tracking your weight, put the scale away for the next 28 days. Instead, let your measure of success be how many days in a row you can do something for your health. It doesn't have to be 18 consecutive minutes. It doesn't even always have to be one of these workouts. If you miss one, just add a few more reps or sets the next day. Adjust the program to fit your life, and trust yourself to be flexible without giving up. By shifting your focus away from outcomes (weight loss) and toward the process (daily movement), you'll alleviate so much of the pressure you put on yourself.

I like to tell clients to walk a wide enough path toward their goals so that when something gets in the way, as it always does, they have other ways to make progress. Realize as you're lying in bed that you missed your workout? That's OK. Instead of stressing, take five deep, mindful breaths at that moment, count

HYDRATION HACKS

Water is essential to success on any fitness plan, but consuming enough is easier said than done. Try these tips to boost hydration all day.

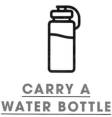

CARRY A WATER BOTTLE

It's especially important in places where you wouldn't likely sit down for a glass of water, such as the grocery store or the car on your morning commute.

EAT FOR HYDRATION

If your job makes it difficult to keep a bottle at hand during the workday, prioritize watery fruits and veggies to stay hydrated. Bonus points for choosing foods with potassium (such as bananas and avocados), which helps prevent dehydration by supporting good fluid balance in your body.

ADD SOME FLAVOR

If you're uninspired to sip plain water all day, try infusing lemon juice or fresh herbs into your glass. Tea is also great, hot or cold, and it can help with afternoon fog or focus issues.

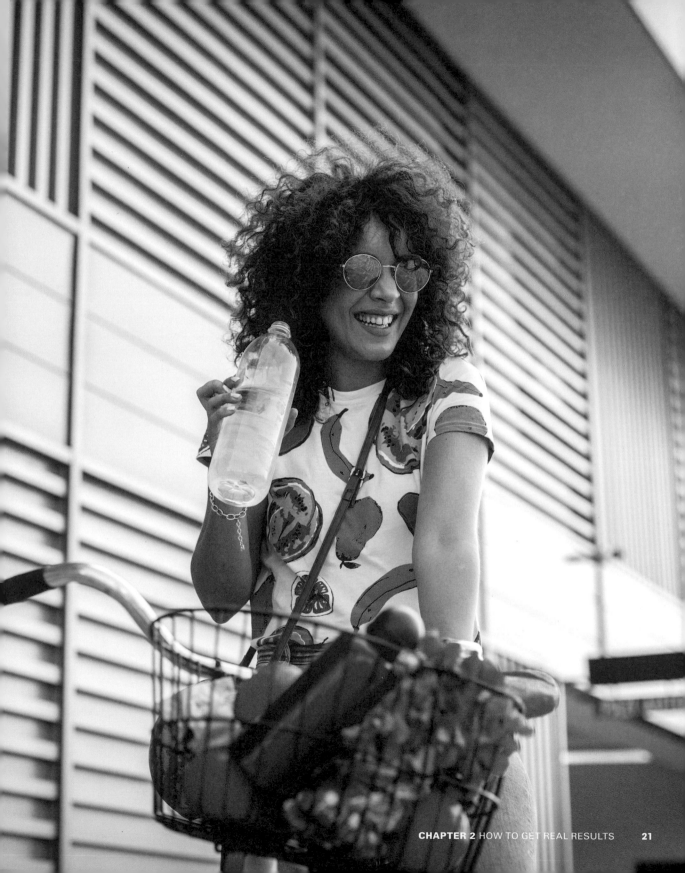

that for the day, and try to do extra reps or sets at your next workout if you have the energy. Take shame, guilt, and perfectionism out of the process. Do not dwell on not being good enough or strong enough or smart enough, or not having the latest workout clothes or gear. Celebrate every single win as often as you can.

FIND YOUR MOTIVATION

Whether you realize it or not, you use motivation to achieve your goals in life. Even if you find enjoyment in an activity, there will be times when you just don't want to get started. Again, widen that path a bit, my friend. Think of one foolproof fun element that you can add to your workout routine for those moments when you'd rather sit on the couch. Maybe you can mark each completed workout day with pretty stickers on a wall calendar. Or budget a reward for yourself, like fresh flowers. Or perhaps you can transform your workout into quality time with someone else: Find a buddy, get your partner or kids involved, hire a trainer. Make your own way of staying consistent! Y'all are free to tag me in your postworkout selfies (@kympossible_fitness on Instagram), and I'll happily celebrate that win with you, if that helps! I personally like to keep sour candies in my gym bag, mostly to help with my asthma while I'm on the stair climber, but also as a little midworkout dopamine boost to do the ab exercises we all put off until the end of the workout. (Yeah, that's right, trainers do that too!)

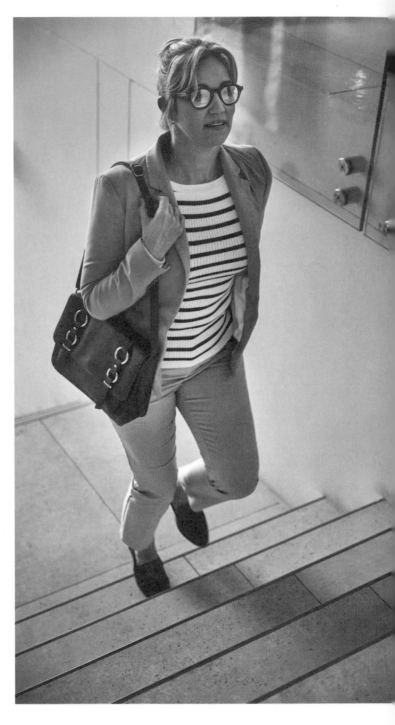

EAT TO SUPPORT YOUR MUSCLES

Just as the right mindset can give your workouts a boost, so can the right foods. To develop and maintain muscle, I suggest you pay attention to generally how much you eat and drink but, more important, to how you feel energywise throughout your day. Focus first on consuming enough protein and water. Your body can't build, preserve, or repair muscle without amino acids, which you can get from protein. Water helps you function at peak performance during your workouts *and* aids in muscle recovery. In terms of how much you need, keep it simple—because measuring or looking up the protein content of foods eventually becomes cumbersome. Instead, try using a visual measurement so you can guesstimate on the go. Aim for a palm-size portion of protein three to four times a day. (That much chicken would be 20 to 30 grams of protein). Your water needs depend on many factors, including how active you are. A good general rule? The classic eight cups is a fine goal, but check in with yourself throughout the day. Feeling thirsty is a sign that you're already a little dehydrated.

Once you've mastered protein and water, think about carbs and fat. These nutrients provide the energy for your workouts and even your mental and emotional state. For carbs, such as brown rice or whole-wheat bread, go for handful-size servings, and keep servings of fat, such as butter or olive oil, to about the size of your thumb pad, or a small spoon. Ultimately, your body will tell you if it needs more of something, so tune in! If your muscles feel heavy, you probably need some protein. Brain fog usually signals a need for carbs, while mood swings can indicate that you need more fat.

FIND LITTLE WAYS TO MOVE

As I mentioned, this 28-day plan was developed so you can see real change without spending your life in the gym. The key to burning more calories outside of your workouts is: 1.) build muscle; and 2) do things that support NEAT, a.k.a. non-exercise activity thermogenesis. NEAT is all the movement you get in your day that *isn't* your workout—such as taking the stairs instead of the elevator, walking the dog, carrying in the groceries, even doing household chores. All of these actions use way more energy than you think and can add up quickly, mostly because your brain is focused on the task, not the reason. Essentially, try to be active! Look for ways to get up and move throughout your day, whether that means setting a timer on your phone to remind you to stand up every 30 minutes, or parking farther from the entrance to your job so you get a few more steps in.

RELAX LIKE IT'S PART OF THE PLAN

Between your workouts and all the NEAT you'll be doing, you'll need to get adequate rest so your muscles can recover and get stronger. That begins with sleep. Quality shut-eye not only gives you the energy you need to bring your A game to your workouts, but also supports muscle growth. And remember: More muscle equals more calories burned at rest. One study found that depriving people of a single night's sleep decreased muscle protein synthesis—the process by which your body builds and repairs muscle mass—by 18%! Try to log seven to nine hours a night. If you're having trouble nodding off, cut out afternoon caffeine and wrap up your screen time at least two hours before bed. Both can make

GET YOUR BEST SLEEP!

Try these simple changes to transform your zzz's.

- Maintain a consistent wake time and bedtime.

- Get daily physical activity.

- Dim the lights two hours before bed.

- Skip alcohol three to four hours before bed.

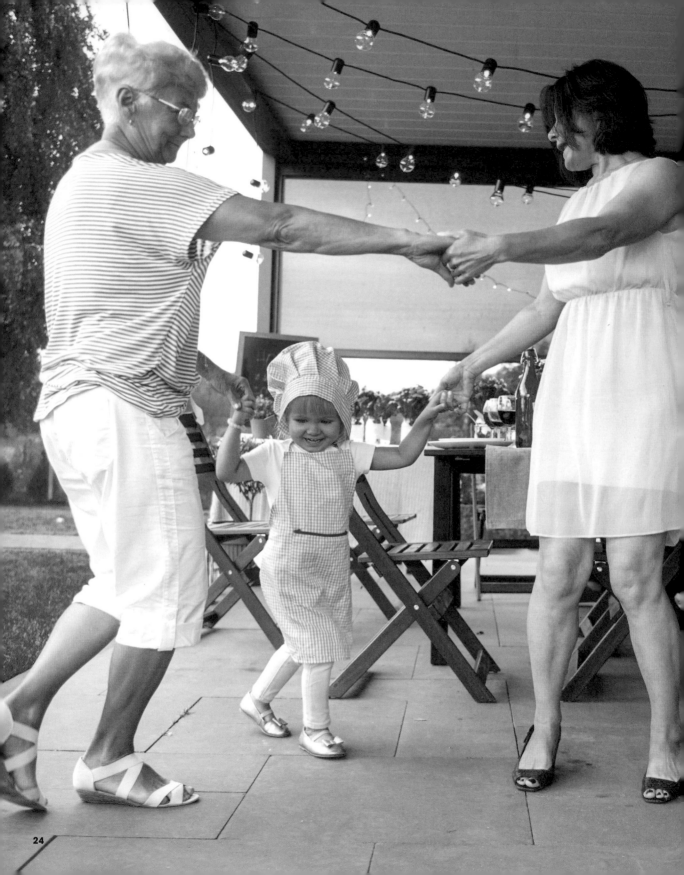

it harder to fall asleep.

Recovery is also vital to your body's muscle-building processes. When you're consistently stressed, your body shifts all of its attention to dealing with the stress. That means other processes, like repairing and building muscle, get deprioritized. Not ideal. In today's high-stress culture, you may be feeling the squeeze from all angles: work deadlines, bills, busy schedules. While some of these stressors may be out of your control, you can work on how you respond to them. My top suggestion? Therapy. It's not just for folks with trauma, and it doesn't necessarily need to involve some major revelation. The goal can simply be to give yourself another tool to address your pain. For me, sometimes it's just about having a place to express my feelings that doesn't feel burdensome to family and friends. Aside from therapy, doing things you enjoy and getting your body moving can help ease stress. I've designed your 28-day plan with these activities built in. Some days your activity will simply be dancing or playing a board game with your family. These relaxing activities are just as crucial to your success in this program as squats and pull-aparts, so make them a priority.

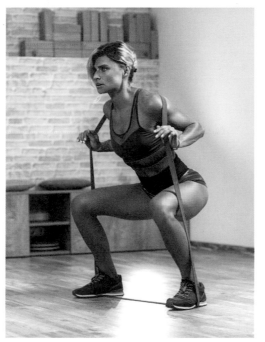

FOCUS ON FORM

Want to know one of the biggest secrets to getting major results from your workouts? It's not doing reps until your arms fall off or hitting the gym for hours every day. It's acing your form. You'll get more out of 12 perfectly executed reps than 25 sloppy ones. When you maintain the correct form as you perform an exercise, you'll activate the correct muscles, which can mean the difference between getting strong abs from crunches or just getting a really strong neckache.

I'm a quality-over-quantity kinda gal, so my suggestion is to take things slow—especially if you're new to exercise, coming back from an injury, or dealing with any kind of chronic pain. As you try the exercises in this plan, move at a moderately slow pace, or at least go slightly slower on the "stretch" part of an exercise, such as lowering yourself down during a push-up. This pace will benefit you in two ways. First, you'll burn more calories by increasing your "time under tension"—meaning you'll be working more of your muscle during a longer period of time per rep and per set. Second, you'll reduce your injury risk by moving a little more slowly than you may want to but also more mindfully. When you tune in to the sensation of each moment of an exercise, you'll be more likely to notice pain arising *before* it leads to injury.

In the exercise glossary, you'll notice that each description indicates which body part you'll be working. This is the body part you should feel engage during the move. Don't worry if sensation comes and goes, but try to focus your attention on that specific area. Move as fully in that range as you can without pain. You might experience a warming sensation in your muscles, and that's normal, though it can definitely feel uncomfortable. Pain is the no-go zone. The reason

Make showing up your top priority. Chances are you'll feel inspired to give a little more than you thought you had once you grab your bands.

I want you to pay attention to specific body parts is because it's common due to being inactive or from injury to accidentally engage the wrong body parts during an exercise and injure yourself. For example, I've had many clients over-rely on their quads rather than using their hamstrings and glutes while completing a squat. This can cause pain and discomfort in your knees. A trick to remember here is that in order to move any part of your body, another part needs to stabilize. If you're moving and feel a little pinch, try creating more stability, like packing your shoulders down a bit.

MAKE THE PLAN YOUR OWN

Life can be unpredictable, so I've designed this program to be adjustable. Each week, you'll see seven different workouts. I've included them in a particular order, but that's just a suggestion. You can follow it exactly if

that's what makes this doable for you, but if that kind of specificity stresses you out, don't worry! Instead, on any given day, you can select the workout that addresses what you feel your body needs that day. The goal is to complete all your workouts for the week, in whatever order.

When I'm scheduling workouts for my clients and myself, I take a glance at the week ahead and generally set what days I want to do what workouts. As the week unfolds, I pay attention to how my body is feeling and what it needs, and then determine if something needs adjusting. For example, say you have a work assignment that's keeping you at the office late. When you get home, you somehow find the will to work out, but you're too tired to cook so you eat a less-than-nourishing dinner. The next morning you wake up exhausted and moody. Your body is telling you it needs more rest, more nutrition, and to regulate your emotions after yesterday. So skip the strength workout and pick the lighter activity for that day. Too often we blame ourselves for not being able to "keep up" in these situations and instead of cutting ourselves some slack, we throw in the towel. But if you widen your path, you'll see that these situations don't need to throw you off course. They can simply guide you in a different direction, one where a stroll around the neighborhood will count as your daily movement. This is how you create healthy habits that can persist even when life gets in the way.

You can customize this plan in other ways. Feel free to change up the time of day when you exercise. If you find yourself wanting more, you can always do another round or combine two days. You can even split your daily 18 minutes into two sessions. Each week of the plan, you'll learn new variations of the exercises from the week before, but go at your own pace. Repeat Week 1 if the moves don't quite feel familiar yet. Or, if you dislike a variation, swap in one that makes you feel good and strong.

However you personalize the plan, make showing up your top priority. Chances are you'll feel inspired to give a little more than you thought you had once you grab your bands.

Find Your "Why"

Identifying the real reason you want to start this fitness journey can help you stay motivated even when sticking to the plan feels impossible. Use this space to reflect on why you want to make this change and revisit it when you're in need of a little motivation to keep going.

I WANT TO START THIS PLAN BECAUSE...

_____

_____

_____

_____

_____

_____

_____

_____

BY THE END OF THIS PLAN, I WANT TO FEEL...

_____

_____

_____

_____

_____

_____

_____

_____

_____

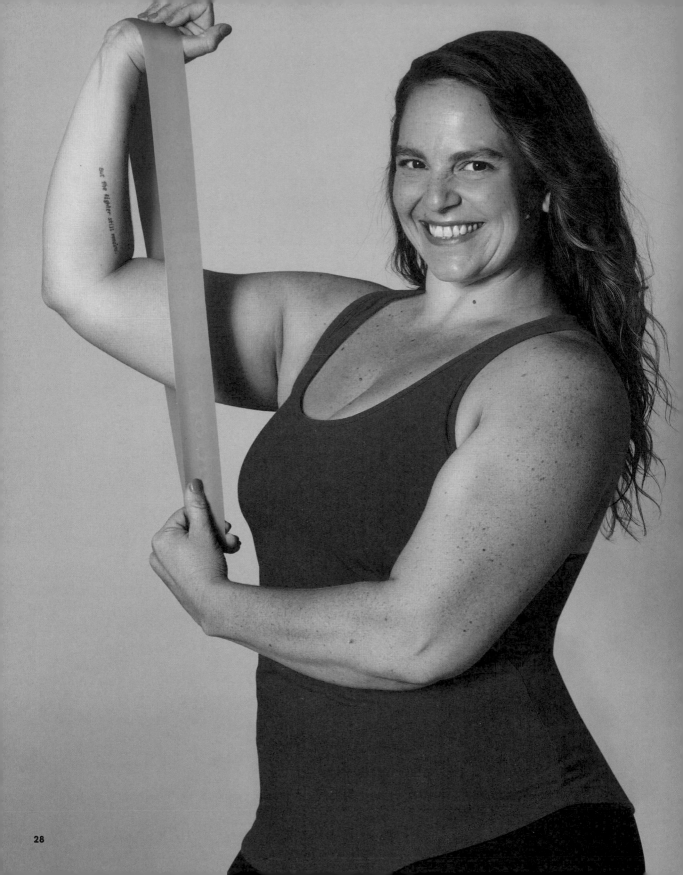

03

Your 28-Day Workout Plan

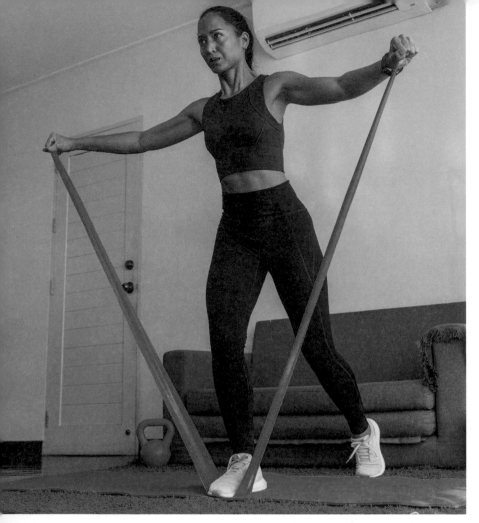

That's actually all the time you need to see results, according to Peter Bregman, the author of *18 Minutes: Find Your Focus, Master Distraction, and Get the Right Things Done*. Bregman found that after 100 hours of practicing, folks actually hit the 95 percentile of skill proficiency. Break 100 hours down into 365 days, and you're left with about 18 minutes a day. Sounds much more manageable than the standard regimen (hour-long workouts, two or three days a week) that you may have tried in the past, right? During those 18 minutes, you'll hit everything from your core to your arms. And none of the exercises require getting down on the ground, making them extra joint-friendly.

As for the number of days you'll follow this plan, start with 28. Building a new habit can take anywhere from 18 to 254 days, according to a study in the *European Journal of Social Psychology*. That's a vast range! So I suggest starting with four solid weeks of work. After those four weeks, you'll begin to build the habit of moving every day. Your body wants what it consistently gets—so before you know it, daily movement will be second nature to you. If you can stack your 18 minutes onto something you already do daily, like watching the morning news or taking the dog out, following the plan can be even easier.

Your weekly routine is also designed to be as stress-free as possible, so you'll find it simple to maintain. Each week builds on the previous one, allowing you to progress at your own pace. Read on for what to expect.

Have you had trouble sticking with exercise routines in the past? I'm confident that you'll be able to keep up with the plan laid out in this chapter. Here's why: For starters, you'll never have to spend more than 18 minutes on your training.

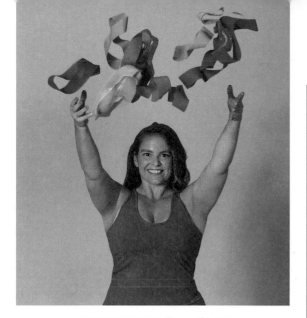

TYPES OF WORKOUTS

**Each week of the plan includes
a mix of the following:**

RESISTANCE TRAINING WORKOUTS

CARDIO WORKOUTS

TOTAL-BODY RESET WORKOUTS

This variety will allow you to work your entire body while also giving your muscles time to rest and recover. You'll also support your cardiovascular health, mobility, and flexibility. And although you'll see a workout listed for each day of the week, this plan is not about pushing beyond your limits. Your cardio, total-body reset, and active NEAT days are more about getting into the habit of setting aside time for movement each day, and they should feel restorative so you can hit your resistance band days with even more energy.

Resistance Training Workouts

These are where you'll be doing all your muscle-building work. If 18 minutes sounds like a lot, don't worry: The workouts are broken into bite-size chunks, with rest built in. You'll complete two circuits, each lasting nine minutes. Each circuit consists of three exercises. Start with three sets of each exercise, and then eventually work your way to a maximum of five sets. You'll do each move for 40 seconds; then you'll have 20 seconds to get into position for the next move. When you've completed all the exercises in the circuit, rest for 45 to 60 seconds before you start back at the top with the first exercise again. This setup allows for the most flexibility. Best of all, you don't have to count reps. Just set a timer on your phone and go!

Your resistance training workouts are further broken down into three types:

Light Resistance Training Days
During these sessions, you'll be doing the lightest amount of strength training. You'll focus more on improving the way your body moves. That doesn't mean you won't be challenged, but these workouts can be an opportunity to move a little more slowly.

Moderate Resistance Training Days
The second resistance training workout you'll do each week, these sessions involve more active movements than your Light Resistance Training days, allowing you to up your intensity a notch.

All Out Resistance Training Days
To round out your week of workouts, you'll perform your most challenging set of exercises and give it your all!

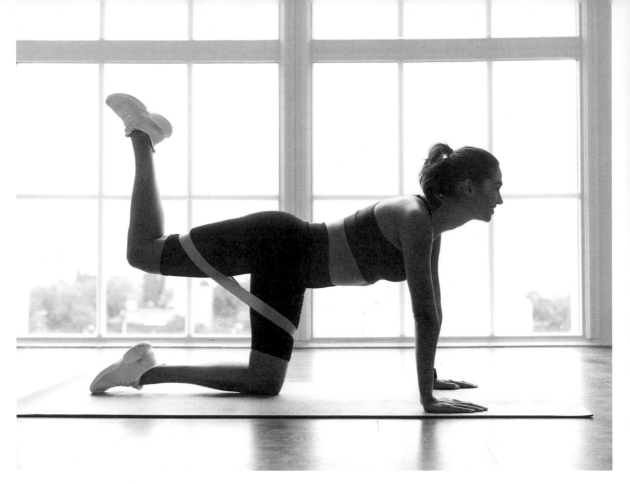

To make it easy to perfect your form and optimize your results, you'll focus on just a handful of key moves in this program. In Week 1, you'll learn a variety of basic exercises. In each week that follows, you'll learn a slightly more challenging variation of each type of exercise. For example, in Week 1 you'll learn the "Level 1" exercise isometric YTWs in which you hold your arms in several different static positions. In Week 2, your "Level 2" variation of the exercise is YTW circles. Here your arms follow a similar pattern but this time you'll move them in circles.

I did this for a few reasons. First, I wanted to make sure you never have to learn an entirely new exercise before feeling comfortable with what's already on your plate. You'll keep honing your technique on these few basic moves the entire program. But you'll never feel bored! Each level offers enough variety to keep you

engaged. The levels are also intended to show you how easy it is to vary resistance band exercises, and how you can build your own workouts well beyond the 28 days.

Here's one more bonus for you: I've organized the exercises in these workouts for maximum efficiency. You'll do your tougher moves earlier in the session in order to rev up a metabolic response that temporarily increases testosterone. You might associate testosterone strictly with men, but everyone needs some. It's especially important for bone and muscle health. This response is useful during your workouts, as it helps you utilize your body's energy efficiently, giving you the push you need to get through a tough set. Plus, completing your more challenging moves at the start of your workout means you'll wrap things up with easier exercises and finish strong.

WHAT YOU'LL NEED

For best results as you complete this program, you'll want to have a variety of resistance bands and loops. (Technically, though, all these moves can be done with just your body weight if needed.) Some bands work best for specific exercises. You may be able to use a long band as a loop by tying its ends, but this can decrease its lifespan, so it's best to buy the right band for the job.

I'm sharing here what I carry with me for my clients and myself. Resistance bands are often sold in packs with three to four different strength levels, which is all you really need. All these exercises are designed to be done standing or sitting, so a chair that allows about a 90-degree bend in your knees is nice, but not necessary.

These are the sizes and types of bands I recommend having in your toolbox or gym bag:

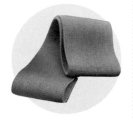	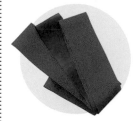	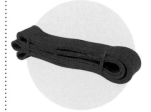	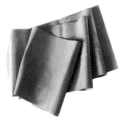
FABRIC MINI LOOP (light and medium)	**ELASTIC MINI LOOP** (light, medium, and hard)	**LONG LOOP** (light, medium, and hard)	**OPEN END LONG BAND** (medium)
I find fabric feels more comfortable and less likely to roll during exercises where the band is looped around my thighs.	Elastic bands tend to be a little thinner than fabric ones, making them ideal for sliding under the arches of your feet or between your toes without adding too much bulk.	Either fabric or rubber bands work here, so buy whichever you prefer.	Some exercises, such as good mornings, are easier with an open band. This style is typically available only in elastic.

Cardio Workouts

Here's where you'll get your heart rate going and that extra calorie burn in. We'll toggle between two different levels of cardio workouts:

Cardio Days

These lighter sessions are all about moving at a steady, consistent pace—whether during a long walk in nature or an afternoon in a museum with a friend. I'll give you ideas for how to spend each day.

Cardio+ Days

Think of these like your regular cardio days but with an added boost! Sometimes you'll do familiar cardio, like walking, but switch between a fast and slow pace, while other times you'll move through a set of high-energy exercises, like mountain climbers and boxing jabs. You'll get your heart rate up a little high, and have fun in the process!

For these days, you'll have a general time-based goal—but the exact activity you do to hit those goals is up to you! I've included example activities for each of these workouts, but the list isn't exhaustive. If it gets you moving and brings you joy, do it! Just aim to do something for at least 18 minutes. Feel free to break up your activity into, say, 10 minutes in the morning and 8 minutes in the evening. It's the daily, consistent practice of moving your body that matters most. Everything else is icing on the cake!

Total-Body Reset Workouts

Finally, I'm giving you my personal body reset routine. This is your big sigh of relief for the week. It includes a series of gentle, feel-good moves to ease you into the next week of the program. This routine can be adjusted to your mood. If you need something more restful, you

can take these moves nice and slow to really relax into the motion. Or, if you're feeling ready to take on a little more, you can make it harder by performing each move for longer or deepening your engagement. By that I mean finding the push and pull in each position. Take the first lunge stretch on page 173: The push is through both feet and the straightening of your back leg. The pull is pulling your hips down and wide to sit your hips as low as you can, bending your front knee, and lengthening your back leg behind. Here's another way to get even more out of this series: Stretch as far as you can in a position, then add an isometric contraction by engaging the muscles you feel stretching and while you think about about using them to pull yourself deeper on every exhale. Inhale to relax a bit without losing the depth, and then exhale as slowly as you can, using the muscles you feel stretching to ever so slightly pull you deeper into the stretch.

You'll get other chances to reset throughout your week and burn calories while you're at it as well. These sessions don't require following a set list of exercises and are an opportunity to add more fun to your fitness routine!

Active NEAT Days

This is your time to do all the little things, like cheering in the stands at a sporting event or even playing a board game, that aren't considered a workout but require movement—and rev up your metabolism. Unlike your cardio and resistance days, your active NEAT days won't get your heart rate pumping or require you to challenge your muscles with a resisting force. These days are simply about reinforcing the habit of being active. Enlist a family member or friend to join you and log some quality social time while you're at it. If you're not sitting completely still, it counts!

Warmups and Cooldowns

It's important to prepare your body for movement so you can avoid injury. However, learning a whole new set of exercises just to warm up isn't always in the cards. So for your warmup, I suggest completing the first three moves of the workout you'll be doing without bands. Do the warmup exercises for as long as the workout charts indicate or less. This allows you to pay extra attention to the way your body feels going through the entire range of motion of an exercise, and also gives you time to adjust your form before incorporating the resistance band. This minimizes the number of new exercises you need to learn, giving you room to focus on the moves in the circuit. Once you're warmed up, do the same three moves with the band along with the rest of the workout.

Cooling down is even more important in my view, especially if you have a lot of stress in your life. It can be a bit jarring to your nervous system to bounce around from life to workout to kids and pets running around. Give yourself even just five minutes to ease the transition from exercise to real life by doing the first sequence in the Total-Body Reset at the end of every workout. This will not only help your body start the recovery process but also gently shift your mindset back into life mode.

What to Do After 28 Days

As mentioned, it takes about 28 days to *begin* to build a habit. To truly solidify your new lifestyle, you have to keep at it. You can repeat the program as is, or continue adjusting it to fit your life. So, yes, this is a 28-day guidebook. However, I hope you can now see that these 28 days are just the beginning phase you can use to build a lifestyle that helps you feel your best while allowing space for you to be human.

Finally, I'll leave you with some simple logic to keep in mind. The more mobile a body gets, the more active that body has the potential to be, and the more likely that body will choose to be active. Focus on what you can do, in this moment, to help yourself feel better. Stop ignoring your body's cues in order to fit someone else's idea of "healthy," and instead listen to what your body is really asking for. Most of the time, especially when it comes to cravings, our bodies want comfort, attention, or security. With this program I hope to encourage you to create a path that feels safe for your body and is centered around addressing your needs first. After that, all you have to do is watch your goals practically achieve themselves. Progress becomes inevitable when the process matches the functionality of *your* body. **You know your body. The more you practice listening to it, the better you'll get at hearing what it needs.**

The 28-Day Plan At A Glance

WEEK 1

Monday	Light Resistance Training 1
Tuesday	Cardio
Wednesday	Moderate Resistance Training 1
Thursday	Cardio+
Friday	All Out Resistance Training 1
Saturday	Active NEAT
Sunday	Total-Body Reset

WEEK 2

Monday	Light Resistance Training 2
Tuesday	Cardio
Wednesday	Moderate Resistance Training 2
Thursday	Cardio+
Friday	All Out Resistance Training 2
Saturday	Active NEAT
Sunday	Total-Body Reset

WEEK 3

Monday	Light Resistance Training 3
Tuesday	Cardio
Wednesday	Moderate Resistance Training 3
Thursday	Cardio+
Friday	All Out Resistance Training 3
Saturday	Active NEAT
Sunday	Total-Body Reset

WEEK 4

Monday	Light Resistance Training 4
Tuesday	Cardio
Wednesday	Moderate Resistance Training 4
Thursday	Cardio+
Friday	All Out Resistance Training 4
Saturday	Active NEAT
Sunday	Total-Body Reset

Week 1: MONDAY

LIGHT RESISTANCE TRAINING 1

	Exercise	Work	Rest	Sets	Notes
	Isometric YTWs p.73	40 sec.	20 sec.	3	
	Single-Arm Diagonal Pushes p.79	40 sec. per side	20 sec.	3	
	Pull-Aparts p.85	40 sec.	20 sec.	3	

COMPLETE ONE SET OF ALL THREE EXERCISES, THEN REST 45–60 SEC.
REPEAT FOR A TOTAL OF THREE SETS.

	Exercise	Work	Rest	Sets	Notes
	Kickstand RDLs p.87	40 sec. per side	20 sec.	3	
	Standing Kickbacks p.93	40 sec. per side	20 sec.	3	
	Pallof Presses p.95	40 sec.	20 sec.	3	

COMPLETE ONE SET OF ALL THREE EXERCISES, THEN REST 45–60 SEC.
REPEAT FOR A TOTAL OF THREE SETS.

Water ⬚ ⬚ ⬚ ⬚ ⬚ ⬚ ⬚ ⬚   **Sleep**
Bedtime Last Night: _____
Wake Time This Morning: _____

Mood _____

Week 1: TUESDAY

CARDIO

Exercise	Work	Notes
Pick one of the following: Walking Jogging Cycling Swimming Hiking	Go for at least 5-10 minutes (or a maximum of 40 minutes) at a slightly elevated state.	

Water ▢▢▢▢▢▢▢▢   **Sleep**
Bedtime Last Night: _____
Wake Time This Morning: _____

Mood _____

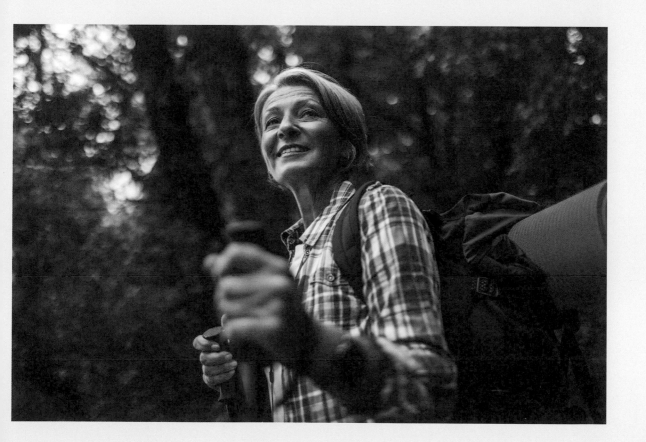

Week 1: WEDNESDAY

MODERATE RESISTANCE TRAINING 1

	Exercise	Work	Rest	Sets	Notes
	"W" Pulls p.101	40 sec.	20 sec.	3	
	Wall Scaptions p.107	40 sec.	20 sec.	3	
	Pull-Aparts p.113	40 sec.	20 sec.	3	

COMPLETE ONE SET OF ALL THREE EXERCISES, THEN REST 45-60 SEC.
REPEAT FOR A TOTAL OF THREE SETS.

	Exercise	Work	Rest	Sets	Notes
	Good Mornings p.119	40 sec.	20 sec.	3	
	Marching p.125	40 sec.	20 sec.	3	
	Chops p.131	40 sec. per side	20 sec.	3	

COMPLETE ONE SET OF ALL THREE EXERCISES, THEN REST 45-60 SEC.
REPEAT FOR A TOTAL OF THREE SETS.

Water ☐☐☐☐☐☐☐☐ **Sleep** **Mood** _____

Bedtime Last Night: _____

Wake Time This Morning: _____

Week 1: THURSDAY

CARDIO+

Exercise	Work	Notes
Pick one of the following: Walking Jogging Cycling Swimming Hiking Playing with a dog or child	Alternate between moving fast and slowing down/resting. For example, walk at your typical pace for 2 minutes, then power walk for 1 minute. Repeat for a total of 18 minutes.	

Water ☐ ☐ ☐ ☐ ☐ ☐ ☐ ☐

Sleep
Bedtime Last Night: _____
Wake Time This Morning: _____

Mood _____

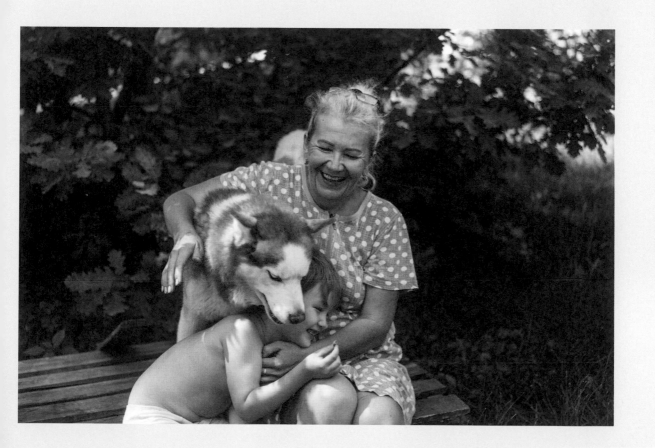

Week 1: FRIDAY

ALL OUT RESISTANCE TRAINING 1

	Exercise	Work	Rest	Sets	Notes
	Isometric Shoulder Abductions p.133	40 sec. per side	20 sec.	3	
	Chest Flys p.139	40 sec.	20 sec.	3	
	Single-Arm Bent-Over Rows p.145	40 sec. per side	20 sec.	3	

COMPLETE ONE SET OF ALL THREE EXERCISES, THEN REST 45-60 SEC. REPEAT FOR A TOTAL OF THREE SETS.

	Exercise	Work	Rest	Sets	Notes
	Squats With Pull-Aparts p.152	40 sec.	20 sec.	3	
	Hip Airplanes p.157	40 sec. per side	20 sec.	3	
	Standing Ab Curl Pull-Downs p.159	40 sec.	20 sec.	3	

COMPLETE ONE SET OF ALL THREE EXERCISES, THEN REST 45-60 SEC. REPEAT FOR A TOTAL OF THREE SETS.

Water ⬜⬜⬜⬜⬜⬜⬜⬜ **Sleep** **Mood** _____
Bedtime Last Night: _____
Wake Time This Morning: _____

Week 1: SATURDAY

ACTIVE NEAT

Exercise	Work	Notes
Pick one of the following: Dancing Doing a family activity Taking a fitness class	Spend as much time as you can with yourself or your family.	

Water ☐☐☐☐☐☐☐☐

Sleep
Bedtime Last Night: _____
Wake Time This Morning: _____

Mood _____

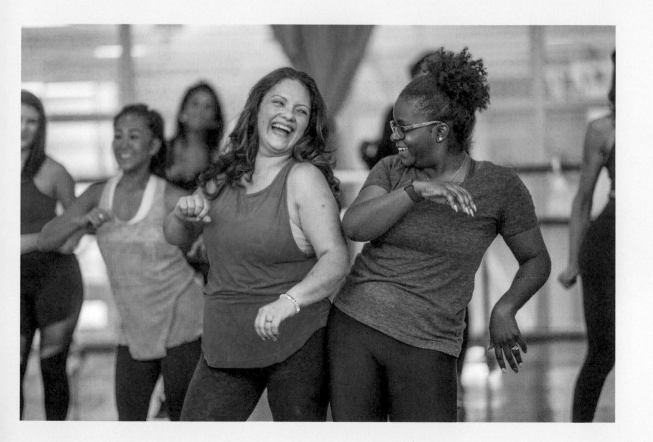

Week 1: SUNDAY

TOTAL-BODY RESET

	Exercise	Work	Notes
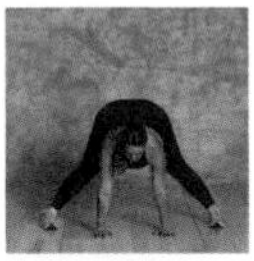	**Triangle Lunge Series** p.173	5 minutes minimum but can be extended to be as long as you need.	
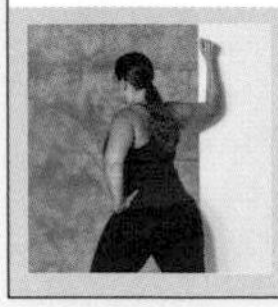	**Doorway Upper-Body Stretch** p.174	5 minutes minimum but can be extended to be as long as you need.	

Water ⬜⬜⬜⬜⬜⬜⬜⬜

Sleep
Bedtime Last Night: _____
Wake Time This Morning: _____

Mood _____

NOTES

Week 2: MONDAY

LIGHT RESISTANCE TRAINING 2

	Exercise	Work	Rest	Sets	Notes
	YTW Circles p.74	40 sec. per position	20 sec.	3	
	Bilateral Low to High Pushes p.80	40 sec.	20 sec.	3	
	Pull-Aparts p.85	40 sec.	20 sec.	3	

COMPLETE ONE SET OF ALL THREE EXERCISES, THEN REST 45-60 SEC. REPEAT FOR A TOTAL OF THREE SETS.

	Exercise	Work	Rest	Sets	Notes
	Rear Foot Elevated RDLs p.88	40 sec. per side	20 sec.	3	
	Standing Kickbacks p.93	40 sec. per side	20 sec.	3	
	Pallof Hold p.96	40 sec.	20 sec.	3	

COMPLETE ONE SET OF ALL THREE EXERCISES, THEN REST 45-60 SEC. REPEAT FOR A TOTAL OF THREE SETS.

Water ☐☐☐☐☐☐☐☐

Sleep
Bedtime Last Night: _____
Wake Time This Morning: _____

Mood _____

Week 2: TUESDAY

CARDIO

Exercise	Work	Notes
Pick one of the following: Cleaning your house Doing yard work	Make a playlist of your favorite songs to listen to while doing chores. Aim to go for a little longer than last week's cardio workout, doing a maximum of 40 minutes.	

Water ⬜⬜⬜⬜⬜⬜⬜⬜

Sleep
Bedtime Last Night: _____
Wake Time This Morning: _____

Mood _____

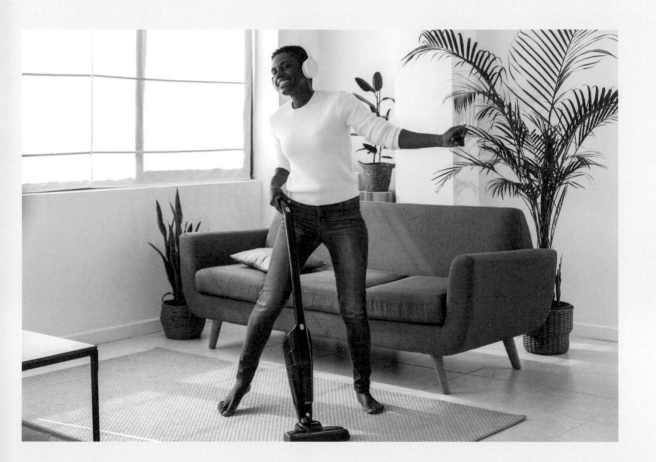

Week 2: WEDNESDAY

MODERATE RESISTANCE TRAINING 2

	Exercise	Work	Rest	Sets	Notes
	Shoulder Flossing p.102	40 sec. per side	20 sec.	3	
	Elevated Banded Push-Ups p.110	40 sec.	20 sec.	3	
	Pull-Aparts Low/High p.114	40 sec.	20 sec.	3	

COMPLETE ONE SET OF ALL THREE EXERCISES, THEN REST 45-60 SEC.
REPEAT FOR A TOTAL OF THREE SETS.

	RDLs p.120	40 sec.	20 sec.	3	
	Step-Ups p.126	40 sec. per side	20 sec.	3	
	Chops p.131	40 sec. per side	20 sec.	3	

COMPLETE ONE SET OF ALL THREE EXERCISES, THEN REST 45-60 SEC.
REPEAT FOR A TOTAL OF THREE SETS.

Water ☐☐☐☐☐☐☐☐

Sleep
Bedtime Last Night: _____
Wake Time This Morning: _____

Mood _____

Week 2: THURSDAY

CARDIO+

	Exercise	Work	Rest	Sets	Notes
	Alternating Reverse Lunges With Pull-Aparts p.165	30 sec.	30 sec.	3	
	Mountain Climbers p.166	30 sec.	30 sec.	3	
	Boxing Jabs p.167	30 sec.	30 sec.	3	

COMPLETE ONE SET OF ALL THREE EXERCISES, THEN REST 45-60 SEC. REPEAT FOR A TOTAL OF THREE SETS.

	Exercise	Work	Rest	Sets	Notes
	Lateral Lunges p.168	30 sec. per side	30 sec.	3	
	Pop Squats p.169	30 sec.	30 sec.	3	
	Thrusters p.170	30 sec.	30 sec.	3	

COMPLETE ONE SET OF ALL THREE EXERCISES, THEN REST 45-60 SEC. REPEAT FOR A TOTAL OF THREE SETS.

Water ▢▢▢▢▢▢▢▢ **Sleep** **Mood** _____
Bedtime Last Night: _____
Wake Time This Morning: _____

Week 2: FRIDAY

ALL OUT RESISTANCE TRAINING 2

	Exercise	Work	Rest	Sets	Notes
	Banded Hand Taps p.134	40 sec. per side	20 sec.	3	
	Decrease Elevation Banded Push-Ups p.140	40 sec.	20 sec.	3	
	Bent-Over Reverse Flys p.146	40 sec.	20 sec.	3	

COMPLETE ONE SET OF ALL THREE EXERCISES, THEN REST 45–60 SEC. REPEAT FOR A TOTAL OF THREE SETS.

	Exercise	Work	Rest	Sets	Notes
	Squats With Band Around Shins p.153	40 sec.	20 sec.	3	
	Hip Airplanes p.157	40 sec. per side	20 sec.	3	
	Standing Ab Curl Push-Downs p.160	40 sec.	20 sec.	3	

COMPLETE ONE SET OF ALL THREE EXERCISES, THEN REST 45–60 SEC. REPEAT FOR A TOTAL OF THREE SETS.

Water ⬜⬜⬜⬜⬜⬜⬜⬜

Sleep
Bedtime Last Night: _____
Wake Time This Morning: _____

Mood _____

Week 2: SATURDAY

ACTIVE NEAT

Exercise	Work	Notes
Pick one of the following: Playing family board games Attending a book club	Use as much time as you can for yourself or your family.	

Water ⊽⊽⊽⊽⊽⊽⊽⊽   **Sleep**
Bedtime Last Night: _____
Wake Time This Morning: _____

Mood _____

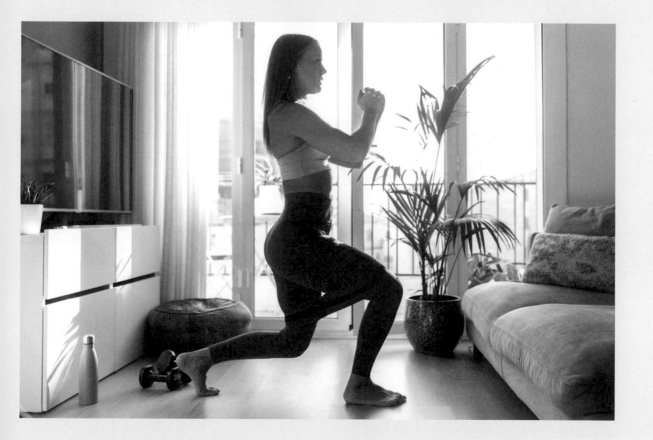

Week 2: SUNDAY

TOTAL-BODY RESET

	Exercise	Work	Notes
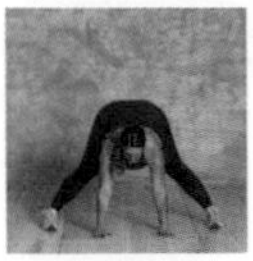	**Triangle Lunge Series** p.173	5 minutes minimum but can be extended to be as long as you need.	
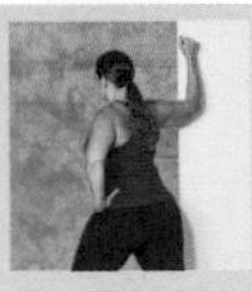	**Doorway Upper-Body Stretch** p.174	5 minutes minimum but can be extended to be as long as you need.	

Water ▢▢▢▢▢▢▢▢

Sleep
Bedtime Last Night: _____
Wake Time This Morning: _____

Mood _____

NOTES

Week 3: MONDAY

LIGHT RESISTANCE TRAINING 3

	Exercise	Work	Rest	Sets	Notes
	YTW Straight-Arm Pulls p.75	40 sec.	20 sec.	3	
	Alternating Isometric Reverse Flys p.81	40 sec.	20 sec.	3	
	Pull-Aparts p.85	40 sec.	20 sec.	3	

COMPLETE ONE SET OF ALL THREE EXERCISES, THEN REST 45–60 SEC.
REPEAT FOR A TOTAL OF THREE SETS.

	Exercise	Work	Rest	Sets	Notes
	Kickstand RDLs With Single-Arm Rows p.90	40 sec. per side	20 sec.	3	
	Standing Kickbacks p.93	40 sec. per side	20 sec.	3	
	Pallof Lateral Steps p.97	40 sec.	20 sec.	3	

COMPLETE ONE SET OF ALL THREE EXERCISES, THEN REST 45–60 SEC.
REPEAT FOR A TOTAL OF THREE SETS.

Water ▢▢▢▢▢▢▢▢   **Sleep**   **Mood** _____
Bedtime Last Night: _____
Wake Time This Morning: _____

Week 3: TUESDAY

CARDIO

Exercise	Work	Notes
Pick one of the following: Visiting a museum Doing a city walking tour	Explore a museum or take walking tour of a city or town—or create your own tour! Aim to go for a little longer than last week's cardio workout, doing a maximum of 40 minutes.	

Water ☐☐☐☐☐☐☐☐

Sleep
Bedtime Last Night: _____
Wake Time This Morning: _____

Mood _____

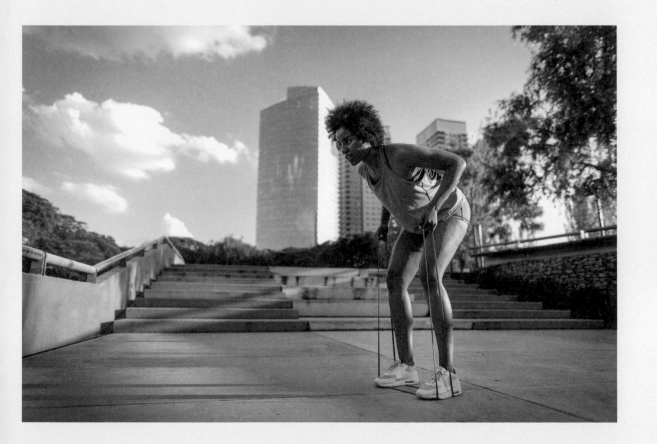

Week 3: WEDNESDAY

MODERATE RESISTANCE TRAINING 3

	Exercise	Work	Rest	Sets	Notes
	Isometric "W" Hold at 90 Degrees p.104	40 sec.	20 sec.	3	
	Decrease Elevation Banded Push-Ups p.109	40 sec.	20 sec.	3	
	Single-Arm Around the Worlds p.116	40 sec. per side	20 sec.	3	

COMPLETE ONE SET OF ALL THREE EXERCISES, THEN REST 45–60 SEC.
REPEAT FOR A TOTAL OF THREE SETS.

	Exercise	Work	Rest	Sets	Notes
	Single-Leg RDLs p.122	40 sec. per side	20 sec.	3	
	Split Squats p.127	40 sec. per side	20 sec.	3	
	Chops p.131	40 sec. per side	20 sec.	3	

COMPLETE ONE SET OF ALL THREE EXERCISES, THEN REST 45–60 SEC.
REPEAT FOR A TOTAL OF THREE SETS.

Water ▯▯▯▯▯▯▯▯   **Sleep**   **Mood** _____

Bedtime Last Night: _____

Wake Time This Morning: _____

Week 3: THURSDAY

CARDIO+

	Exercise	Work	Rest	Sets	Notes
	Alternating Reverse Lunges With Pull-Aparts p.165	30 sec.	30 sec.	3	
	Mountain Climbers p.166	30 sec.	30 sec.	3	
	Boxing Jabs p.167	30 sec.	30 sec.	3	

COMPLETE ONE SET OF ALL THREE EXERCISES, THEN REST 45–60 SEC.
REPEAT FOR A TOTAL OF THREE SETS.

	Exercise	Work	Rest	Sets	Notes
	Lateral Lunges p.168	30 sec. per side	30 sec.	3	
	Pop Squats p.169	30 sec.	30 sec.	3	
	Thrusters p.170	30 sec.	30 sec.	3	

COMPLETE ONE SET OF ALL THREE EXERCISES, THEN REST 45–60 SEC.
REPEAT FOR A TOTAL OF THREE SETS.

Water ⬛⬛⬛⬛⬛⬛⬛⬛ **Sleep** **Mood** _____
Bedtime Last Night: _____
Wake Time This Morning: _____

Week 3: FRIDAY

ALL OUT RESISTANCE TRAINING 3

	Exercise	Work	Rest	Sets	Notes
	Shoulder Circles p.135	40 sec.	20 sec.	3	
	Alternating Isometric Chest Flys p.141	40 sec.	20 sec.	3	
	Alternating Single-Arm Bent-Over Rows p.147	40 sec.	20 sec.	3	

COMPLETE ONE SET OF ALL THREE EXERCISES, THEN REST 45–60 SEC.
REPEAT FOR A TOTAL OF THREE SETS.

	Exercise	Work	Rest	Sets	Notes
	Squats With Band Around Shins and Under Big Toes p.154	40 sec.	20 sec.	3	
	Hip Airplanes p.157	40 sec. per side	20 sec.	3	
	Isometric Banded Standing Marching p.161	40 sec.	20 sec.	3	

COMPLETE ONE SET OF ALL THREE EXERCISES, THEN REST 45–60 SEC.
REPEAT FOR A TOTAL OF THREE SETS.

Water ▢▢▢▢▢▢▢▢   **Sleep**   **Mood** _____
Bedtime Last Night: _____
Wake Time This Morning: _____

Week 3: SATURDAY

ACTIVE NEAT

Exercise	Work	Notes
Pick one of the following: Going climbing Playing a seasonal sport Doing a seasonal activity	Use as much time as you can for yourself or your family.	

Water ⬜⬜⬜⬜⬜⬜⬜⬜

Sleep
Bedtime Last Night: _____
Wake Time This Morning: _____

Mood _____

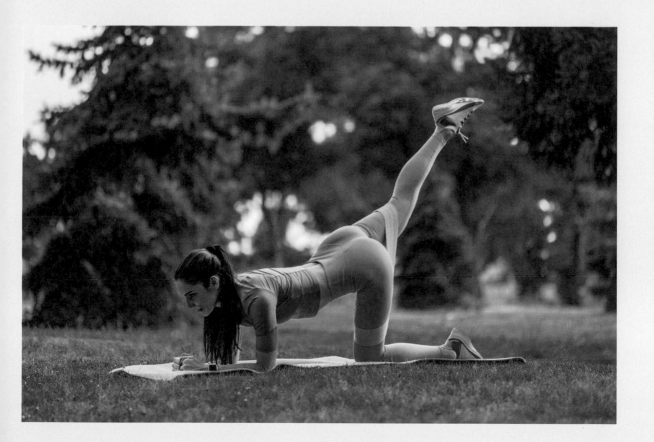

Week 3: SUNDAY

TOTAL-BODY RESET

	Exercise	Work	Notes
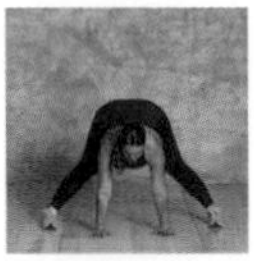	**Triangle Lunge Series** p.173	5 minutes minimum but can be extended to be as long as you need.	
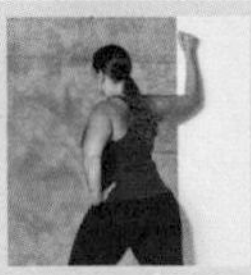	**Doorway Upper-Body Stretch** p.174	5 minutes minimum but can be extended to be as long as you need.	

Water ▭ ▭ ▭ ▭ ▭ ▭ ▭ ▭

Sleep
Bedtime Last Night: _____
Wake Time This Morning: _____

Mood _____

NOTES

Week 4: MONDAY

LIGHT RESISTANCE TRAINING 4

	Exercise	Work	Rest	Sets	Notes
	Standing Internal Rotation Pull-Downs p.76	40 sec. per side	20 sec.	3	
	Standing Isometric Bird Dogs p.82	40 sec. per side	20 sec.	3	
	Pull-Aparts p.85	40 sec.	20 sec.	3	

COMPLETE ONE SET OF ALL THREE EXERCISES, THEN REST 45-60 SEC.
REPEAT FOR A TOTAL OF THREE SETS.

	Exercise	Work	Rest	Sets	Notes
	Rear Foot Elevated RDLs With Single-Arm Rows p.91	40 sec. per side	20 sec.	3	
	Standing Kickbacks p.93	40 sec. per side	20 sec.	3	
	Pallof March p.98	40 sec.	20 sec.	3	

COMPLETE ONE SET OF ALL THREE EXERCISES, THEN REST 45-60 SEC.
REPEAT FOR A TOTAL OF THREE SETS.

Water ▢▢▢▢▢▢▢▢ **Sleep**
Bedtime Last Night: _____
Wake Time This Morning: _____

Mood _____

Week 4: TUESDAY

ACTIVE NEAT

Exercise	Work	Notes
Any type of volunteering: Handing out food or supplies Cleaning your neighborhood Helping out at an animal shelter	Not only can you get plenty of NEAT here but you'll also be doing something for others and that boosts your happy chemicals!	

Water ▢▢▢▢▢▢▢▢

Sleep
Bedtime Last Night: _____
Wake Time This Morning: _____

Mood _____

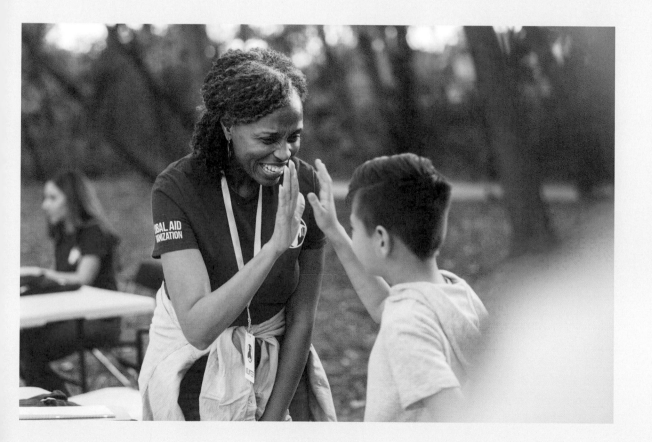

Week 4: WEDNESDAY

MODERATE RESISTANCE TRAINING 4

	Exercise	Work	Rest	Sets	Notes
	Isometric Vertical Abductions p.105	40 sec.	20 sec.	3	
	Elevated Banded Back Push-Ups p.110	40 sec.	20 sec.	3	
	Bilateral Around the Worlds p.117	40 sec.	20 sec.	3	

COMPLETE ONE SET OF ALL THREE EXERCISES, THEN REST 45–60 SEC. REPEAT FOR A TOTAL OF THREE SETS.

	Exercise	Work	Rest	Sets	Notes
	Deadlifts p.123	40 sec.	20 sec.	3	
	Bird Dogs p.128	40 sec. per side	20 sec.	3	
	Chops p.131	40 sec. per side	20 sec.	3	

COMPLETE ONE SET OF ALL THREE EXERCISES, THEN REST 45–60 SEC. REPEAT FOR A TOTAL OF THREE SETS.

Water ☐☐☐☐☐☐☐☐

Sleep
Bedtime Last Night: _____
Wake Time This Morning: _____

Mood _____

Week 4: THURSDAY

CARDIO+

	Exercise	Work	Rest	Sets	Notes
	Alternating Reverse Lunges With Pull-Aparts p.165	30 sec.	30 sec.	3	
	Mountain Climbers p.166	30 sec.	30 sec.	3	
	Boxing Jabs p.167	30 sec.	30 sec.	3	

COMPLETE ONE SET OF ALL THREE EXERCISES, THEN REST 45–60 SEC.
REPEAT FOR A TOTAL OF THREE SETS.

	Exercise	Work	Rest	Sets	Notes
	Lateral Lunges p.168	30 sec. per side	30 sec.	3	
	Pop Squats p.169	30 sec.	30 sec.	3	
	Thrusters p.170	30 sec.	30 sec.	3	

COMPLETE ONE SET OF ALL THREE EXERCISES, THEN REST 45–60 SEC.
REPEAT FOR A TOTAL OF THREE SETS.

Water ⬜⬜⬜⬜⬜⬜⬜⬜   **Sleep**   **Mood** _____
Bedtime Last Night: _____
Wake Time This Morning: _____

Week 4: FRIDAY

ALL OUT RESISTANCE TRAINING 4

	Exercise	Work	Rest	Sets	Notes
	Vertical Shoulder Circles p.136	40 sec.	20 sec.	3	
	Single-Arm Vertical Pushes p.142	40 sec. per side	20 sec.	3	
	Standing Vertical Pull-Downs p.148	40 sec. per side	20 sec.	3	

COMPLETE ONE SET OF ALL THREE EXERCISES, THEN REST 45–60 SEC.
REPEAT FOR A TOTAL OF THREE SETS.

	Exercise	Work	Rest	Sets	Notes
	Squats to Heel Raises With Pull-Aparts p.155	40 sec.	20 sec.	3	
	Hip Airplanes p.157	40 sec. per side	20 sec.	3	
	Isometric Bent-Over Lat Pull-Downs p.162	40 sec.	20 sec.	3	

COMPLETE ONE SET OF ALL THREE EXERCISES, THEN REST 45–60 SEC.
REPEAT FOR A TOTAL OF THREE SETS.

Water ▢▢▢▢▢▢▢▢   **Sleep**
Bedtime Last Night: _____
Wake Time This Morning: _____

Mood _____

Week 4: SATURDAY

ACTIVE NEAT

Exercise	Work	Notes
Pick one of the following: Attending a sporting event Playing a recreational sport	Use as much time as you can for yourself or your family.	

Water ▯ ▯ ▯ ▯ ▯ ▯ ▯ ▯

Sleep
Bedtime Last Night: _____
Wake Time This Morning: _____

Mood _____

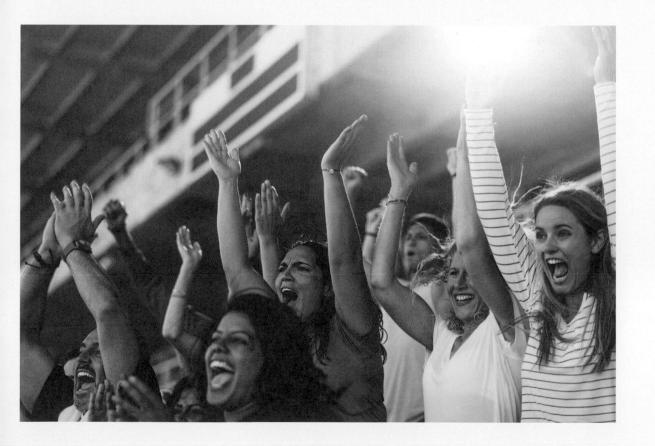

Week 4: SUNDAY

TOTAL-BODY RESET

	Exercise	Work	Notes
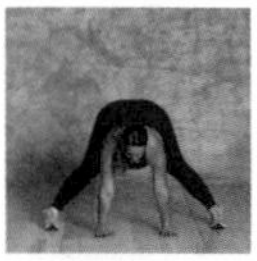	**Triangle Lunge Series** p.173	5 minutes minimum but can be extended to be as long as you need.	
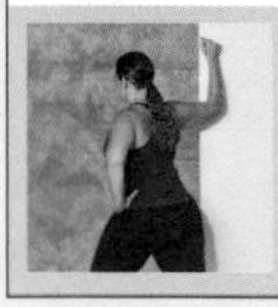	**Doorway Upper-Body Stretch** p.174	5 minutes minimum but can be extended to be as long as you need.	

Water ☐☐☐☐☐☐☐☐

Sleep
Bedtime Last Night: _____
Wake Time This Morning: _____

Mood _____

NOTES

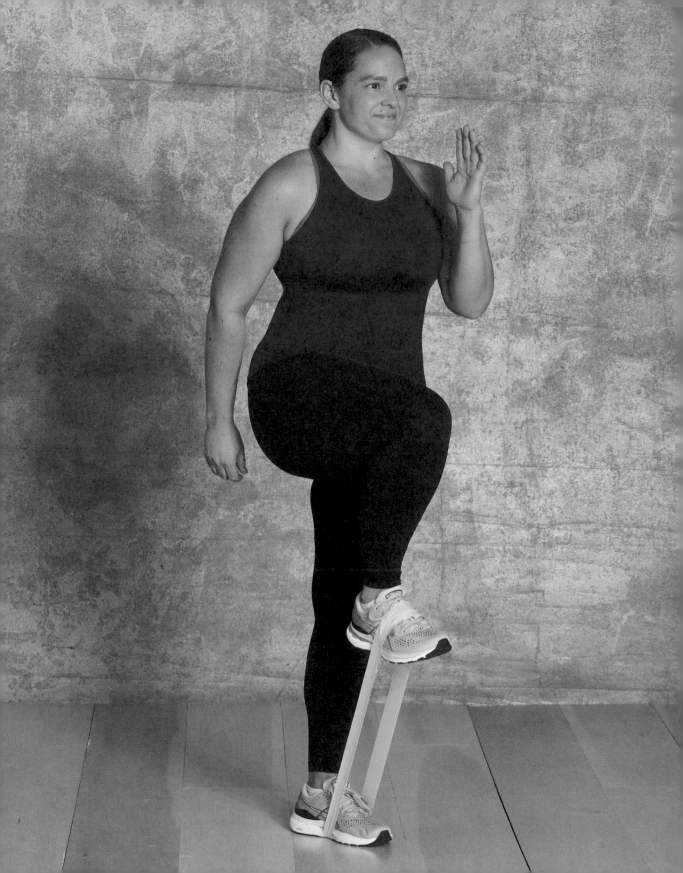

04

Exercise Glossary

Light Resistance Training

Shoulder Exercises

As mentioned earlier, you'll learn a few key moves in the first week of this program, then build upon that foundation every week that follows with slightly more challenging variations of those same moves. In this glossary, those variations are grouped together so you can see how the work you do in Week 1 benefits you in Week 2, 3, and 4 (and beyond!).

The very first exercise you'll do in this plan focuses on your shoulders. Although perhaps not the first body part you think about exercising, strong shoulders are essential to overall fitness. This series taps into the little muscles around your shoulders like those pesky rotator cuffs and deltoids, which can cause posture-related issues and even headaches or numbness in your fingers. If you sit in front of a computer for long periods of time, adding these into your routine can significantly alleviate the aches and pains that result from prolonged sitting. Plus, these movements make it easier to move your shoulders in all directions, which in turn will make it easier to do all kinds of upper-body exercises. As you perform these moves, think about activating your mid-back, shoulders, and arms.

AT A GLANCE

**Level 1:
Isometric YTWs**
p.73

**Level 2:
YTW Circles**
p.74

**Level 3:
YTW Straight-Arm
Pulls**
p.75

**Level 4: Standing
Internal Rotation
Pull-Downs**
p.76

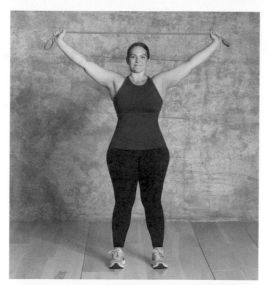

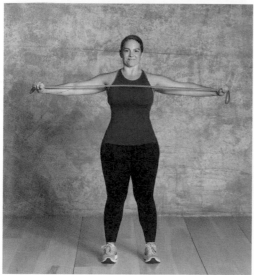

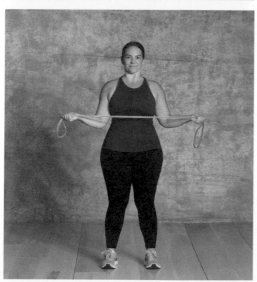

| LEVEL 1 | LEVEL 2 | LEVEL 3 | LEVEL 4 |

ISOMETRIC YTWS

SETUP Stand with feet hip-width apart, holding one end of a long band in each hand.

STEP 1 Inhale to anchor your shoulder blades.

STEP 2 Exhale to raise your arms overhead and slightly wider than your shoulders so your body forms a "Y." Hold for the prescribed amount of time.

STEP 3 Lower your arms out to the sides to shoulder height, forming a "T." Hold for the prescribed amount of time.

STEP 4 Bend your elbows and glue them to your sides to form a "W." Hold for the prescribed amount of time.

STEP 5 Return to the starting position. Continue for the prescribed amount of time.

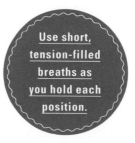

Use short, tension-filled breaths as you hold each position.

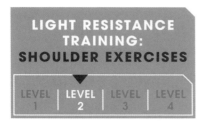

YTW CIRCLES

SETUP Stand with feet hip-width apart, holding one end of a long band in each hand.

STEP 1 Inhale to anchor your shoulder blades.

STEP 2 Exhale to raise your arms overhead and slightly wider than your shoulders so your body forms a "Y." Make tiny circles with your arms for the prescribed amount of time.

STEP 3 Lower your arms out to the sides to shoulder height, forming a "T." Make tiny circles with your arms for the prescribed amount of time.

STEP 4 Bend your elbows and glue them to your sides to form a "W." Make tiny circles with your arms for the prescribed amount of time.

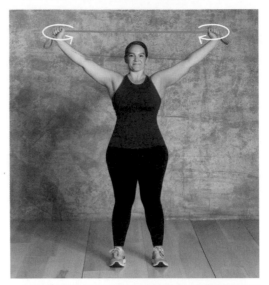

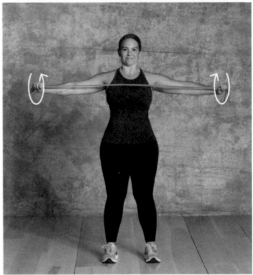

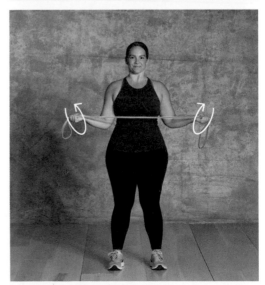

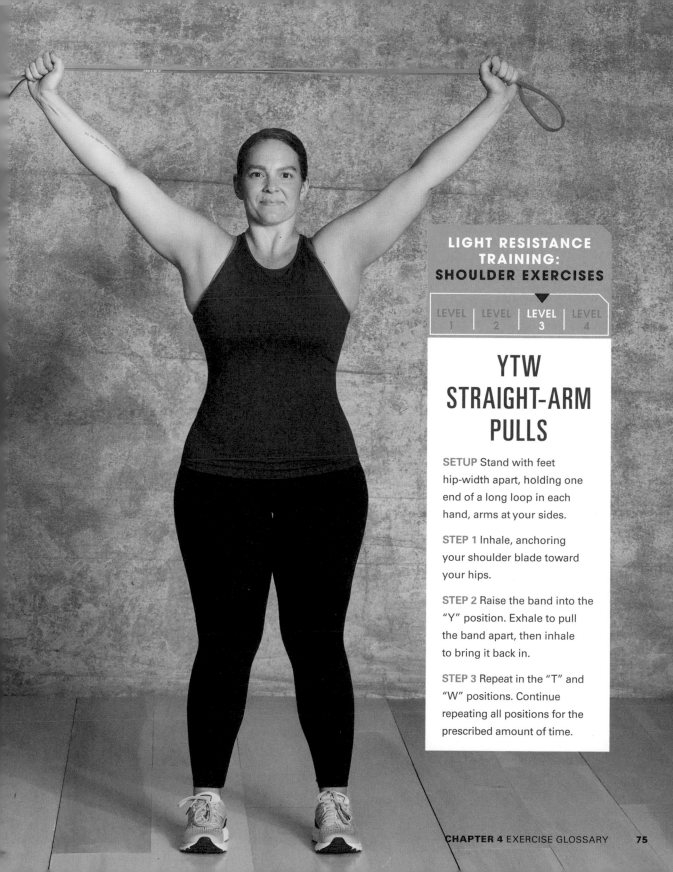

| LEVEL 1 | LEVEL 2 | **LEVEL 3** | LEVEL 4 |

YTW STRAIGHT-ARM PULLS

SETUP Stand with feet hip-width apart, holding one end of a long loop in each hand, arms at your sides.

STEP 1 Inhale, anchoring your shoulder blade toward your hips.

STEP 2 Raise the band into the "Y" position. Exhale to pull the band apart, then inhale to bring it back in.

STEP 3 Repeat in the "T" and "W" positions. Continue repeating all positions for the prescribed amount of time.

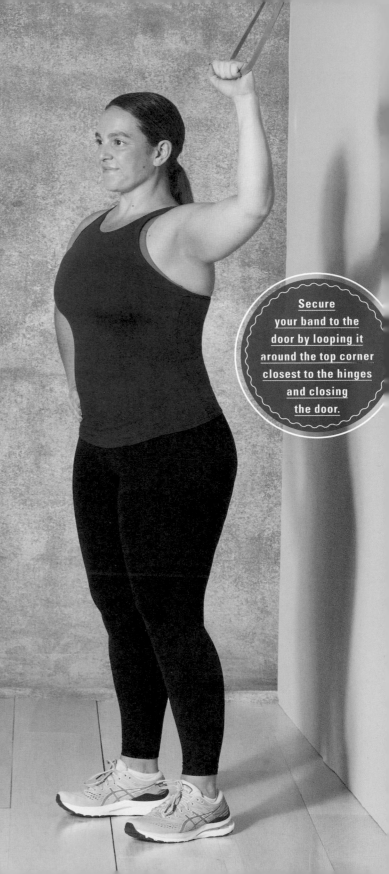

LEVEL 1	LEVEL 2	LEVEL 3	LEVEL 4

STANDING INTERNAL ROTATION PULL-DOWNS

SETUP Anchor a band over top of a door or bar. Stand tall with feet hip distance apart and a few steps facing away from the wall. Hold the end of the band in your left hand, your left elbow about shoulder height out to the side.

STEP 1 Keeping the elbow out at shoulder height, inhale, anchoring the shoulders toward your hips.

STEP 2 Exhale, keeping the elbow shoulder height, pull the band forward toward the floor. Return to the starting position. Continue for the prescribed amount of time then repeat on the opposite side.

Secure your band to the door by looping it around the top corner closest to the hinges and closing the door.

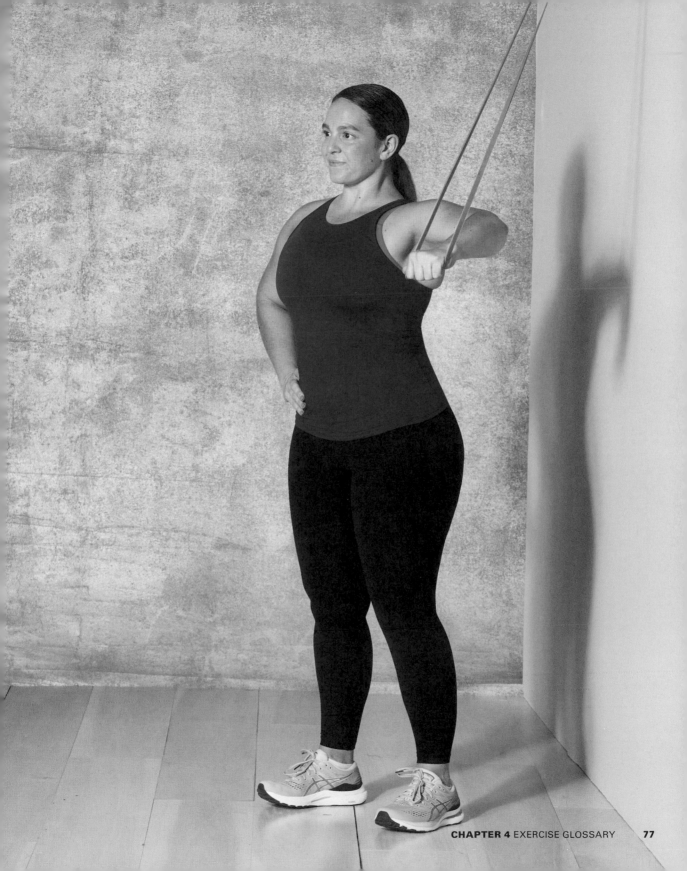

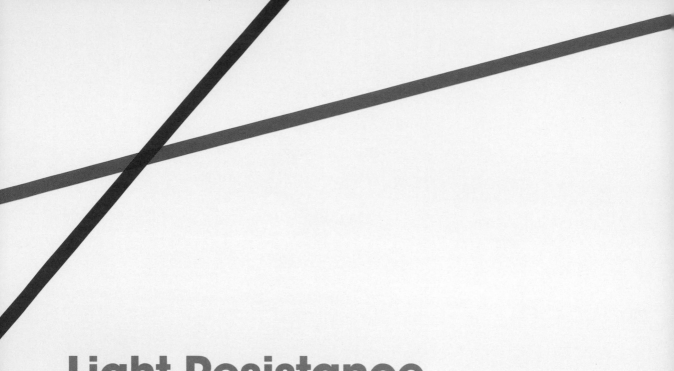

Light Resistance Training

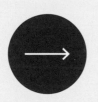

Push Exercises

There are two types of movements that are crucial to strong upper body muscles, posture, and balance: push and pull. It's important to do them both, which is why you'll find movements from this section and the "pull" section (page 84) in each workout. Push exercises are just what they sound like—moves that involve a pushing motion, like pushing the end of a long loop over your head.

For this series, you'll want to focus on building stability. In order to move any part of your body, you have to stabilize—or keep still—another body part. In these exercises, it's your proud chest and shoulder blades that should stay still as you push in various directions. Stabilizing can also help alleviate aches you might experience during an exercise. In the upper body, that usually means anchoring your shoulder blades, which I'll remind you to do throughout this plan.

AT A GLANCE

**Level 1:
Single-Arm
Diagonal Pushes**
p.79

**Level 2:
Bilateral Low to
High Pushes**
p.80

**Level 3:
Alternating
Isometric Reverse
Flys** p.81

**Level 4:
Standing
Isometric
Bird Dogs** p.82

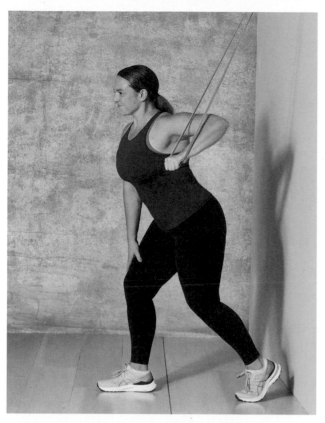

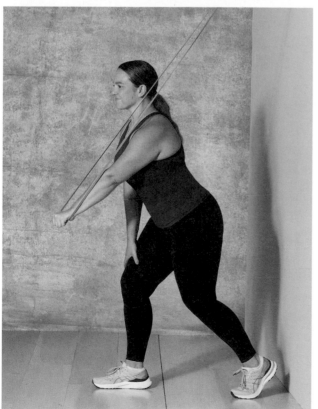

SINGLE-ARM DIAGONAL PUSHES

SETUP Anchor a long band high on a door or bar. Hold the ends in your left hand and turn your body away from the door, stepping your right foot in front. Bring your left hand to the front of your left shoulder, elbow pointing behind you.

STEP 1 Inhale to anchor your shoulder blades toward your hips.

STEP 2 Exhale to push the band at a downward diagonal in front of you. Return to the starting position. Continue for the prescribed amount of time then repeat on the opposite side.

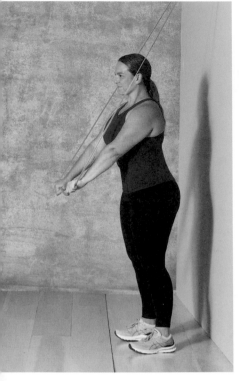
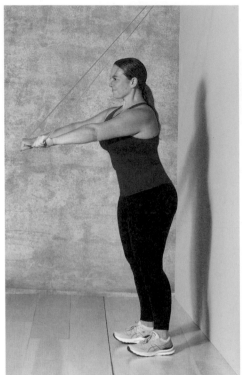
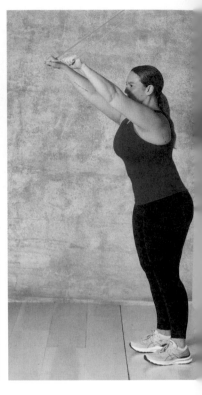

LIGHT RESISTANCE
TRAINING:
PUSH EXERCISES

| LEVEL 1 | LEVEL 2 | LEVEL 3 | LEVEL 4 |

Only go as
high as you can
while keeping
your shoulders
down.

BILATERAL LOW TO HIGH PUSHES

SETUP Anchor a long band high on a door or bar. Hold the ends in both hands and turn your body away from the door.

STEP 1 Inhale to anchor your shoulder blades toward your hips.

STEP 2 Exhale to push the band at a downward diagonal in front of you.

STEP 3 Keep your shoulders anchored as you allow the band to bring your straight arms toward the upward diagonal. Pull your elbows back to return to the starting position. Continue for the prescribed amount of time.

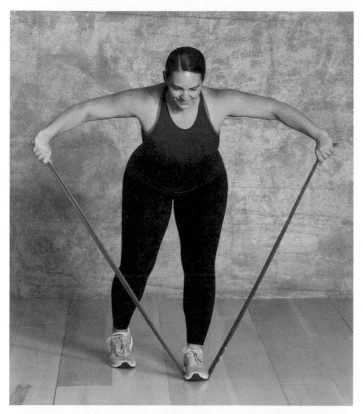

ALTERNATING ISOMETRIC REVERSE FLYS

SETUP Stand with feet hip-width apart and staggered with your left foot in front. Loop a long band under the arch of your left foot, holding one end in each hand.

STEP 1 Inhale to anchor your shoulders toward your hips. Exhale to open your arms like you're about to give someone a hug, squeezing your shoulder blades together behind you.

STEP 2 Lower your right arm.

STEP 3 Raise your right arm back to the starting position.

STEP 4 Lower your left arm.

STEP 5 Raise your left arm back to the starting position. Continue alternating for the prescribed amount of time, using short, tension-filled breaths.

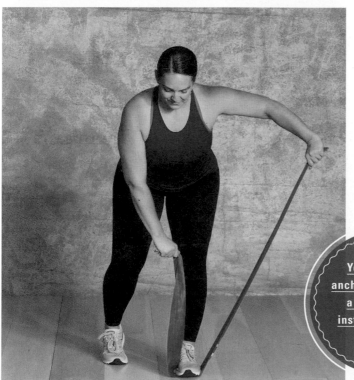

You can also anchor the band to a door or bar instead of under your foot.

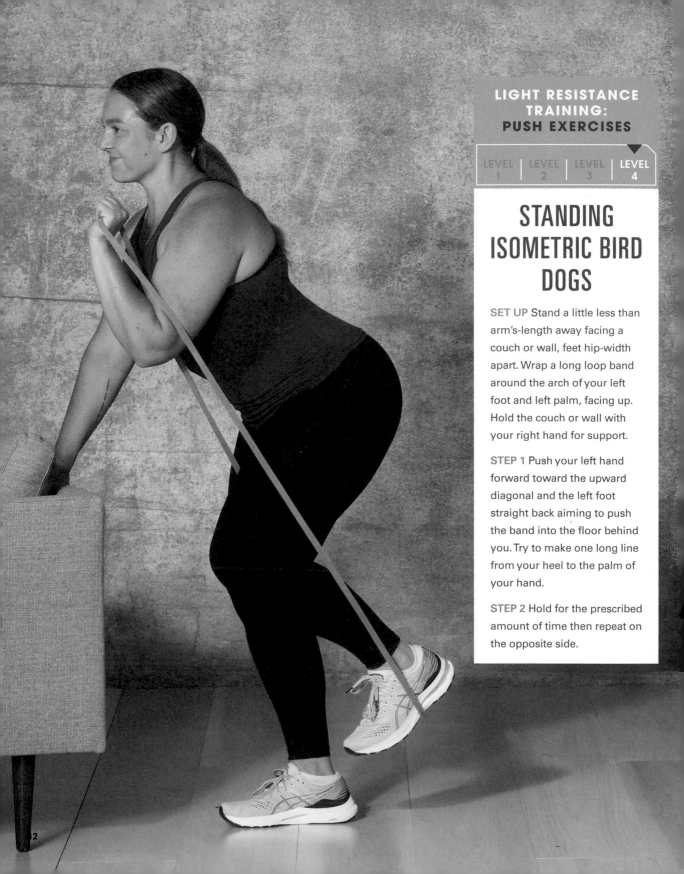

STANDING ISOMETRIC BIRD DOGS

SET UP Stand a little less than arm's-length away facing a couch or wall, feet hip-width apart. Wrap a long loop band around the arch of your left foot and left palm, facing up. Hold the couch or wall with your right hand for support.

STEP 1 Push your left hand forward toward the upward diagonal and the left foot straight back aiming to push the band into the floor behind you. Try to make one long line from your heel to the palm of your hand.

STEP 2 Hold for the prescribed amount of time then repeat on the opposite side.

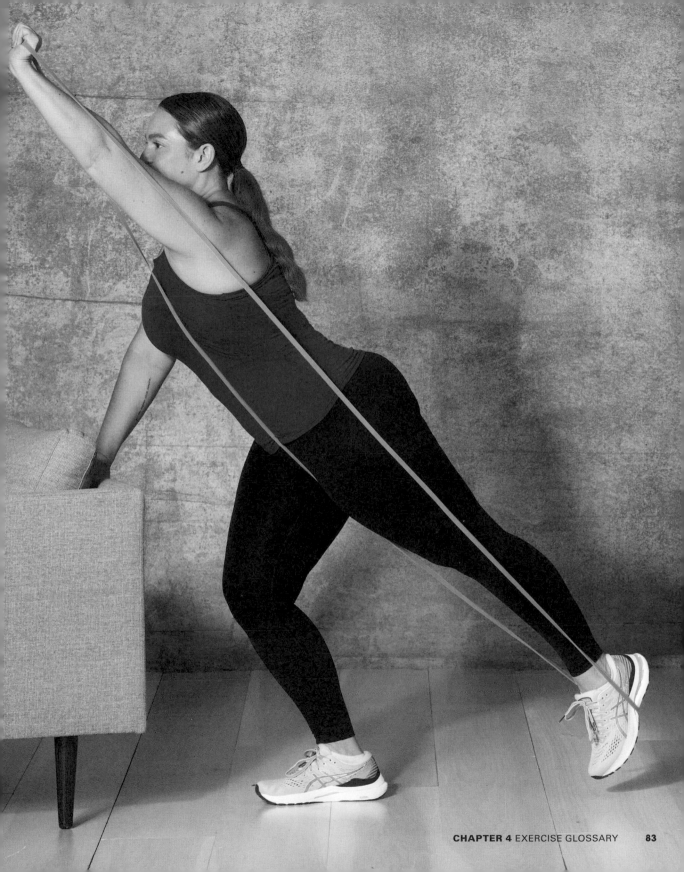

Light Resistance Training

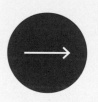

Pull Exercises

To complement the pushing movements in this plan, you'll start with one of the most efficient pull exercises there is: pull-aparts. They're so powerful that they're the only move you'll do for all levels of your Light Resistance Training pull series. The motion is simple—pull the ends of a long band in opposite directions—making them great for beginners. Plus, they're highly effective on their own or tacked on to another exercise, like squats. Try it with a super heavy band for more resistance or add it to a cardio move. You'll see benefits in so many areas, from your posture and breathing functions to your upper-body strength and core functionality.

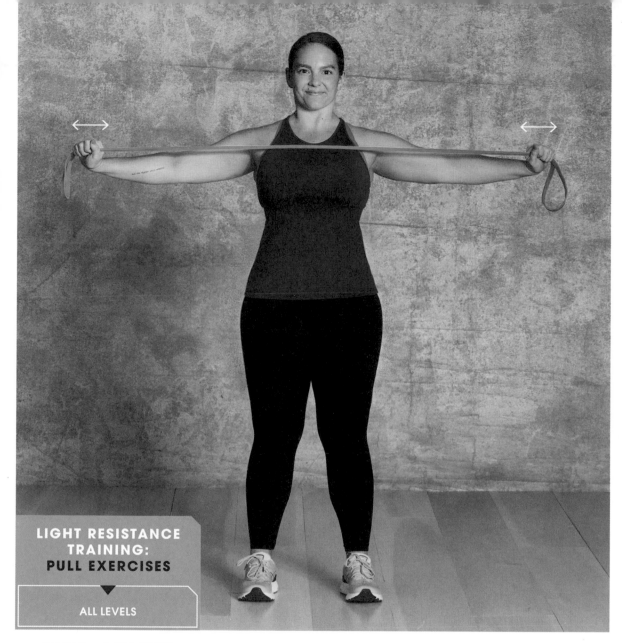

PULL-APARTS

SETUP Stand with feet hip-width apart, arms extended shoulder-width in front of you holding one end of a long band in each hand, palms facing down.

STEP 1 Inhale to anchor shoulder blades down toward your hips.

STEP 2 Exhale and squeeze your shoulder blades together, pulling the band apart with a slight bend in your elbows.

STEP 3 Return to the starting position. Continue for the prescribed amount of time.

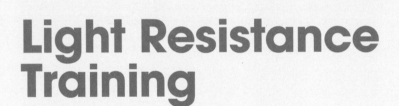

Light Resistance Training

Hip Hinge Exercises

Improving your ability to hinge at the hip will make so many of life's daily to-do's easier. Putting on a pair of pants, bending down to tie a shoe, picking a sock up off the floor—all these actions require a strong hip hinge. This series of exercises are all variations of a Romanian deadlift (RDL) and will help you build just that, plus boost your balance. You'll decrease your risk of falls, move through everyday tasks with less effort, and tone your lower body. To master these moves, aim to keep your hips "square." Think of your hip bones on the front of your pelvis as a car's headlights. You need to keep your headlights pointed straight in front of you in order to stay on the road, so do the same with your hips and you'll be on the path to hip hinge success!

AT A GLANCE

**Level 1:
Kickstand RDLs**
p.87

**Level 2:
Rear Foot
Elevated RDLs**
p.88

**Level 3:
Kickstand RDLs
With Single-Arm
Rows** p.90

**Level 4:
Rear Foot
Elevated RDLs
With Single-Arm
Rows** p.91

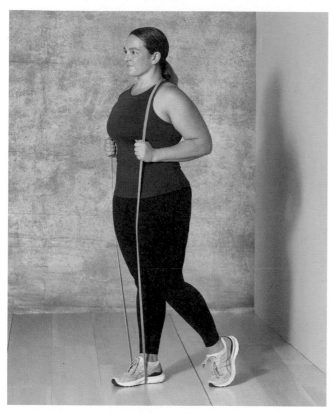

KICKSTAND RDLS

SETUP Stand with feet hip-width apart, a long loop under the arch of your right foot and over your shoulders. Use your hands to hold the band to keep it in a comfortable position across your shoulders.

STEP 1 Shift your head, chest, and hips over your right foot, tucking your left foot back slightly so just your toes are touching the floor, knees in line with each other and hips square.

STEP 2 Inhale, aim to sit your right hip toward your left heel while keeping your weight over your right foot. This creates a slight "swivel" or shift in the hips that helps you to access your right glute. It's not a twist, more a slight shift of the banded hip toward the opposite, lifted heel.

STEP 3 Straighten your legs and stand upright to return to the starting position. Continue for the prescribed amount of time then repeat on the opposite side.

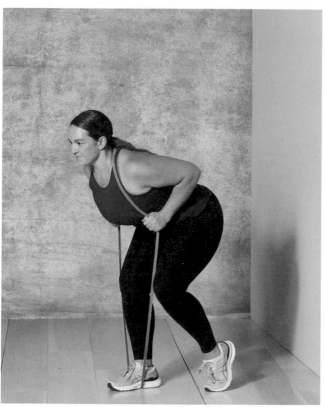

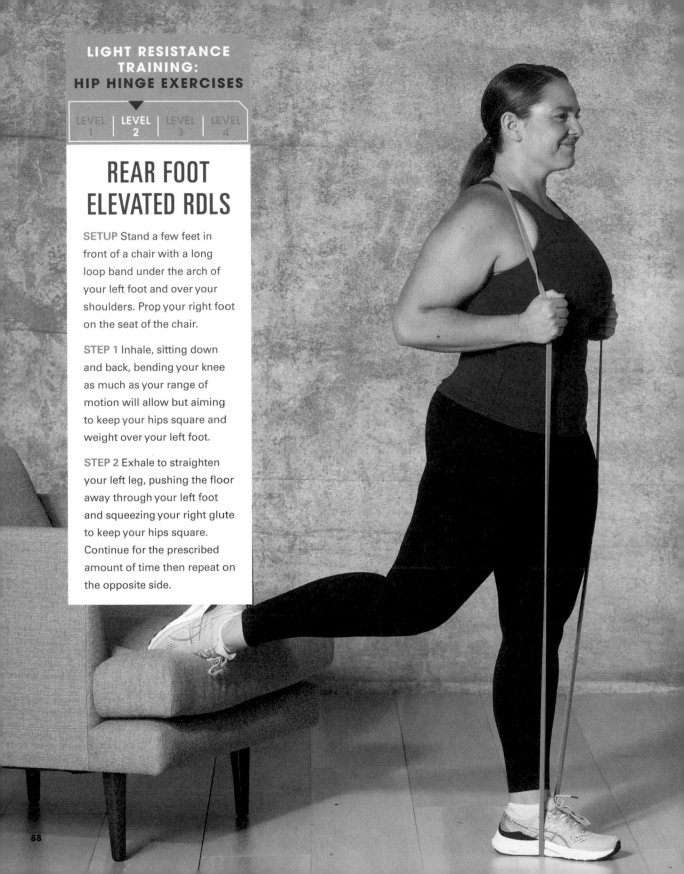

REAR FOOT ELEVATED RDLS

SETUP Stand a few feet in front of a chair with a long loop band under the arch of your left foot and over your shoulders. Prop your right foot on the seat of the chair.

STEP 1 Inhale, sitting down and back, bending your knee as much as your range of motion will allow but aiming to keep your hips square and weight over your left foot.

STEP 2 Exhale to straighten your left leg, pushing the floor away through your left foot and squeezing your right glute to keep your hips square. Continue for the prescribed amount of time then repeat on the opposite side.

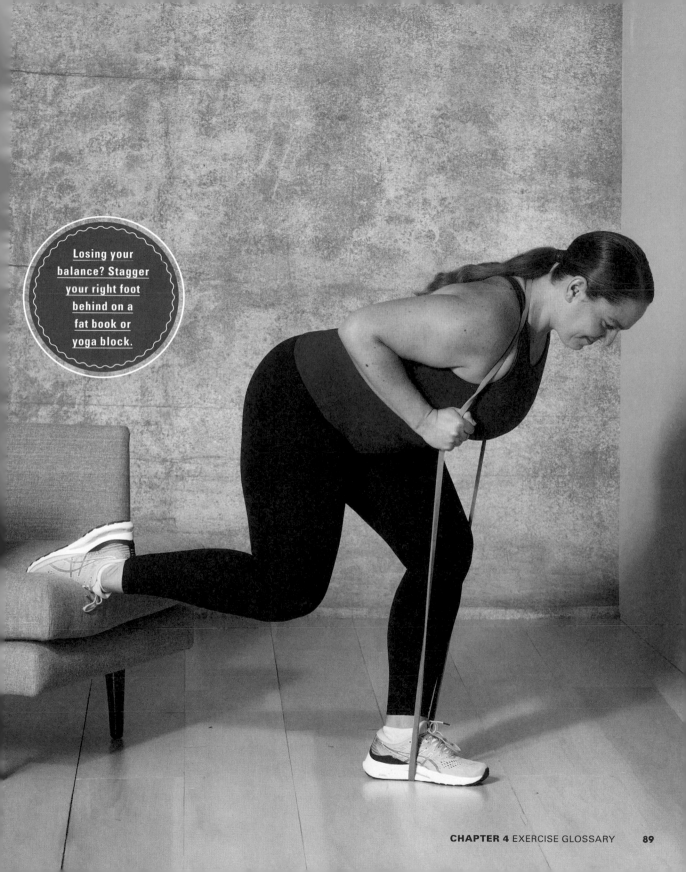

Losing your balance? Stagger your right foot behind on a fat book or yoga block.

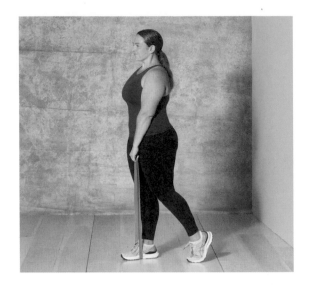

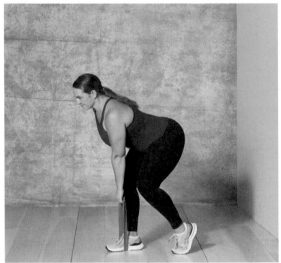

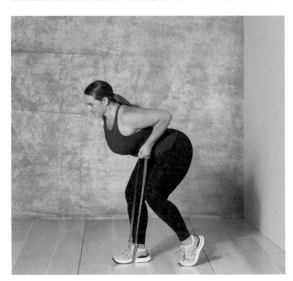

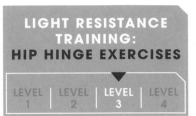

| LEVEL 1 | LEVEL 2 | LEVEL 3 | LEVEL 4 |

KICKSTAND RDLS WITH SINGLE-ARM ROWS

SETUP Stand with feet hip-width apart, one end of a mini loop under the arch of your right foot, the other in your left hand.

STEP 1 Shift your head, chest, and hips over your right foot, tucking your left foot back slightly so just your toes are touching the floor, knees in line with each other and hips square.

STEP 2 Hinge back until your proud chest is about parallel to the ground, your weight remaining over your right foot.

STEP 3 Inhale to anchor your shoulder blades and exhale, driving your left elbow behind you toward the ceiling and aiming your hand to your hip bone. Return your left arm to the starting position. Continue for the prescribed amount of time then repeat on the opposite side.

LEVEL 1	LEVEL 2	LEVEL 3	LEVEL 4

REAR FOOT ELEVATED RDLS WITH SINGLE-ARM ROWS

SETUP Stand a few feet in front of a chair with one end of a mini loop band under the arch of your left foot, the other end in your right hand.

STEP 1 Shift your head, chest, and hips over your left foot, tucking your right foot back slightly so just your toes are touching the floor, knees in line with each other and hips square.

STEP 2 Hinge back until your proud chest is about parallel to the ground, your weight remaining over your left foot.

STEP 3 Raise your back foot onto the seat of the chair.

STEP 4 Inhale to anchor your shoulder blades and exhale, driving your right elbow behind you toward the ceiling and aiming your hand to your hip bone. Lower your arm back down and return to an upright position. Continue for the prescribed amount of time then repeat on the opposite side.

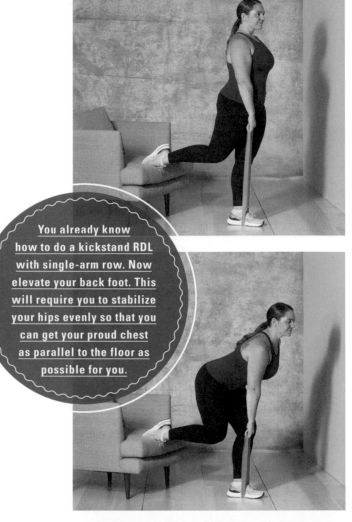

You already know how to do a kickstand RDL with single-arm row. Now elevate your back foot. This will require you to stabilize your hips evenly so that you can get your proud chest as parallel to the floor as possible for you.

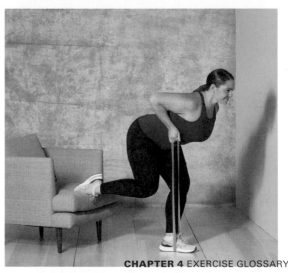

Light Resistance Training

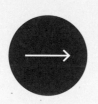

Single-Leg Exercises

In my opinion, there's no better beginner-friendly exercise for toning your lower body and improving your balance than standing kickbacks, so you'll do this move for all levels of this single-leg series. Driving your working leg straight back fires up your glutes, while standing on one leg challenges your balance. To further target your hamstrings, hold a small ball or yoga block between the glute and heel of the working leg. Even though it's called a kickback, think of it as a "lift back" and only lift as high as you can while primarily working your hamstrings and glutes.

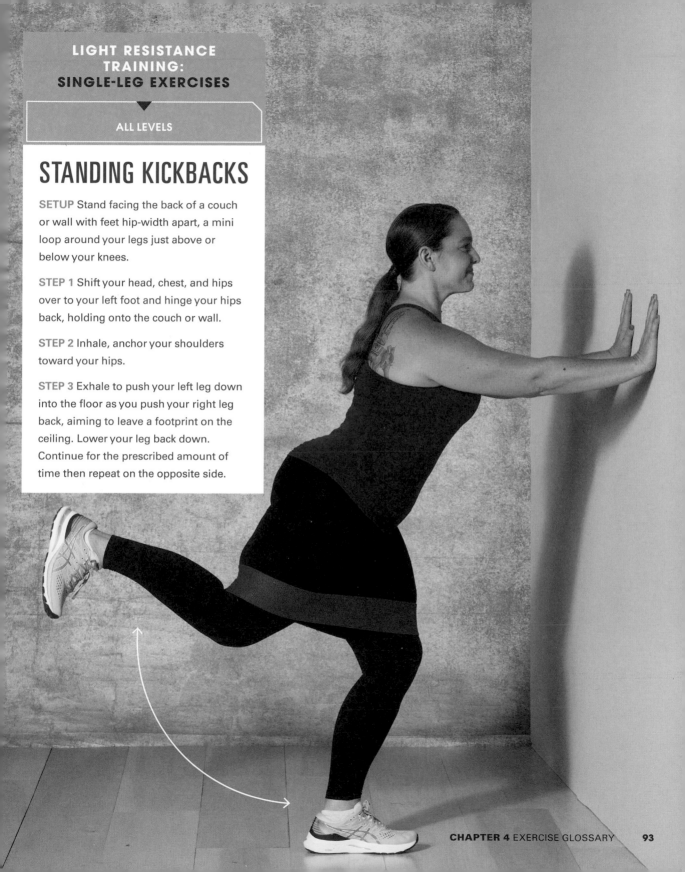

STANDING KICKBACKS

SETUP Stand facing the back of a couch or wall with feet hip-width apart, a mini loop around your legs just above or below your knees.

STEP 1 Shift your head, chest, and hips over to your left foot and hinge your hips back, holding onto the couch or wall.

STEP 2 Inhale, anchor your shoulders toward your hips.

STEP 3 Exhale to push your left leg down into the floor as you push your right leg back, aiming to leave a footprint on the ceiling. Lower your leg back down. Continue for the prescribed amount of time then repeat on the opposite side.

Light Resistance Training

Core Exercises

You don't have to do endless crunches to get a strong core. In fact, the moves in this series will help you build core strength without ever getting on the floor! Not only that, they'll also develop your anti-rotation strength, a.k.a. your ability to resist twisting your torso. It might not sound like a strength you'll utilize often, but it's critical to keep you from toppling over when you may need to scoop up a little one or pet who's running around. It even impacts the simple act of walking. As you walk, your legs and arms move forward and backward, encouraging your torso to turn sideways. Your anti-rotation work prevents you from twisting back and forth with each stride (which would make it pretty hard to get anywhere!). It all adds up to more balanced, stable, and pain-free movement.

AT A GLANCE

Level 1:
Pallof Presses
p.95

Level 2:
Pallof Hold
p.96

Level 3:
Pallof Lateral Steps
p.97

Level 4:
Pallof March
p.98

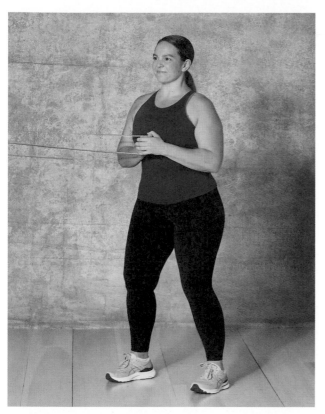

PALLOF PRESSES

SETUP Anchor a long band around a doorknob. Stand with feet slightly wider than hip-width perpendicular to the line of your band, holding the band with both hands at sternum height in the center of your body.

STEP 1 Inhale, anchor your shoulder blades, then exhale and push your hands straight out in front of you without letting the band pull you.

STEP 2 Inhale to pull your arms in, resisting the twisting pull of the band. Continue for the prescribed amount of time.

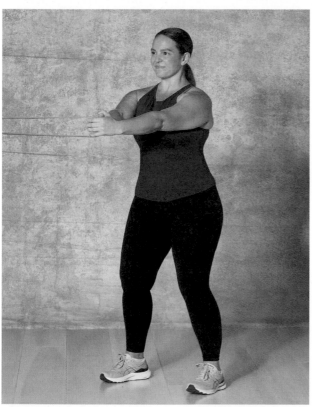

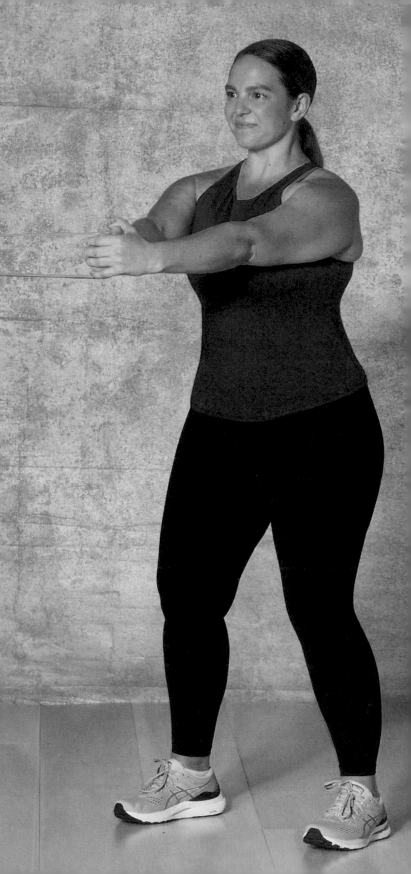

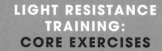

LIGHT RESISTANCE TRAINING: CORE EXERCISES

LEVEL 1	LEVEL 2	LEVEL 3	LEVEL 4

PALLOF HOLD

SETUP Anchor a long band around a doorknob. Stand with feet slightly wider than hip-width perpendicular to the line of your band, holding the band with both hands at sternum height in the center of your body, elbows at your sides.

STEP 1 Inhale, anchor your shoulder blades, exhale to push out as far as you can to maintain your anchored shoulders, then use those short tension-filled breaths to hold for the prescribed amount of time.

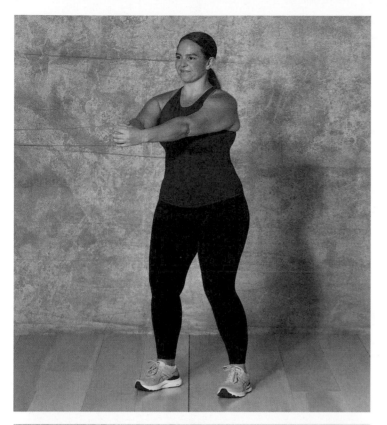

| LEVEL 1 | LEVEL 2 | LEVEL 3 | LEVEL 4 |

PALLOF LATERAL STEPS

SETUP Anchor a long band around a doorknob. Stand with feet slightly wider than hip-width perpendicular to the line of your band, holding the band with both hands at sternum height in the center of your body, elbows at your sides.

STEP 1 Inhale, anchor your shoulder blades, exhale to push out as far as you can maintain your shoulders anchored, then use those short tension-filled breaths to hold.

STEP 2 Take a few small, even steps sideways away from the anchor and back toward, staying square in your body and even in your steps. Continue for the prescribed amount of time.

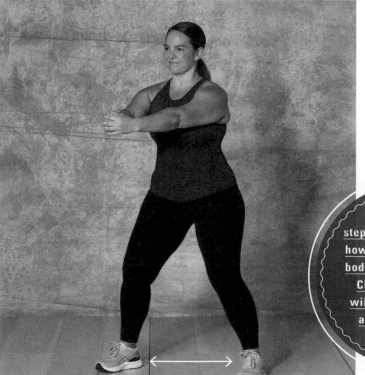

For the lateral steps, you can play with how far away from your body you hold the band. Closer to your body will be easier, farther away will be more challenging.

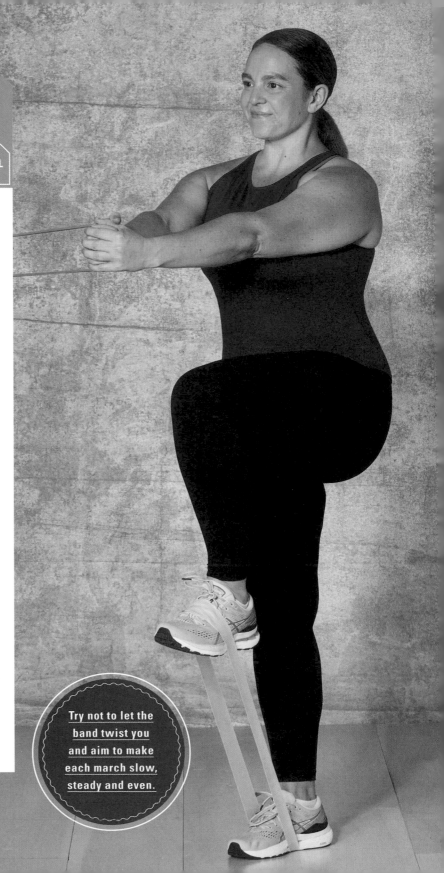

LEVEL 1	LEVEL 2	LEVEL 3	LEVEL 4

PALLOF MARCH

SETUP Anchor a long band around a doorknob, then place a mini loop under the arches of your feet. Hold the long band in both hands at the center of your sternum, elbows at your sides and feet hip-width apart.

STEP 1 Inhale, anchor your shoulder blades, exhale to push out as far as you can maintain your anchored shoulders. Use short tension-filled breaths to continue anchoring your shoulders.

STEP 2 Inhale to shift your head, chest, and hips over your right foot.

STEP 3 Exhale to slowly lift your left knee up, aiming to raise it parallel to the ground by the end of your exhale.

STEP 4 Inhale to return your left leg to the starting position. Repeat on the opposite side. Continue alternating sides for the prescribed amount of time.

Try not to let the band twist you and aim to make each march slow, steady and even.

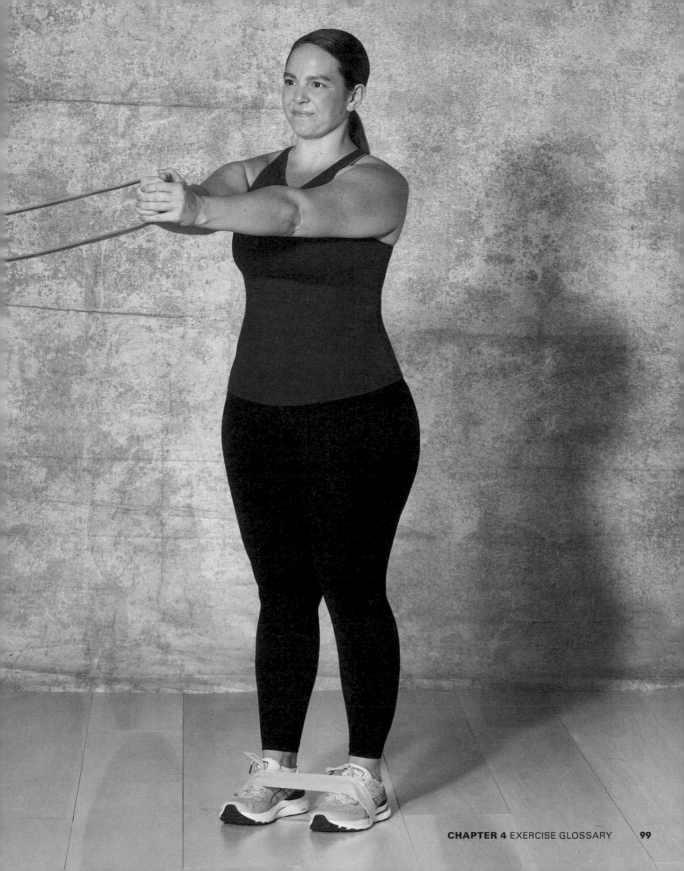

Moderate Resistance Training

Shoulder Exercises

For your second series of shoulder exercises in this plan, you'll continue to build upper body strength while also unwinding tight muscles from long periods of sitting. Most of us spend hours parked in a chair each day hunched forward. Over time this causes the back of your body to overstretch and the front of your body to compact, which all translates to feeling tight. These exercises ease the tension in two ways: They increase mobility in the muscles that are tight and strengthen the muscles that can help prevent tightness in these areas in the first place. To get the most from these moves, focus on activating the muscles in between your shoulder blades as well as the ones that cradle underneath them. In the shoulder flossing exercise, you should also feel a stretch on the front of the shoulder on the same side of the bottom hand.

AT A GLANCE

Level 1:
"W" Pulls
p.101

Level 2:
Shoulder Flossing
p.102

Level 3:
Isometric "W"
Holds at 90
Degrees p.104

Level 4:
Isometric Vertical
Abductions
p.105

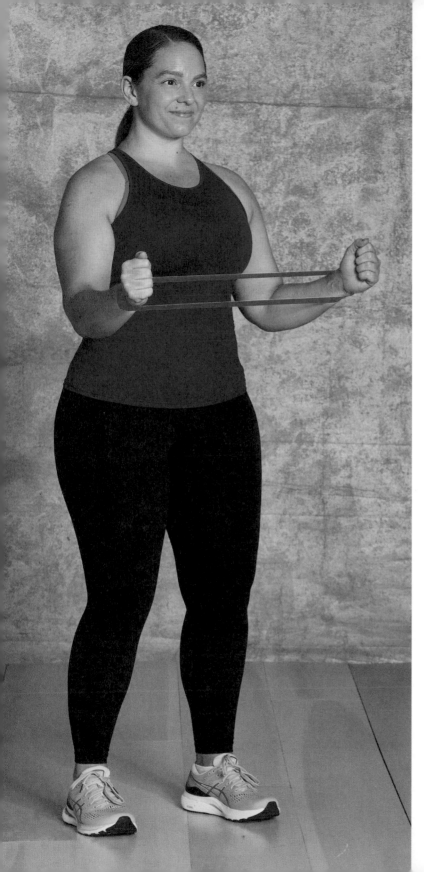

| LEVEL 1 | LEVEL 2 | LEVEL 3 | LEVEL 4 |

"W" PULLS

SETUP Stand with feet hip-width apart, a mini loop around your wrists or holding one end of a long band in each hand, hands facing in and clenched. Glue your elbows to your sides, your forearms parallel to the ground.

STEP 1 Keeping your elbows glued to your sides, inhale and anchor your shoulders down toward your hips.

STEP 2 Exhale, squeezing your shoulder blades together as you pull the band apart.

STEP 3 Inhale to control the movement back to the starting position. Continue for the prescribed amount of time.

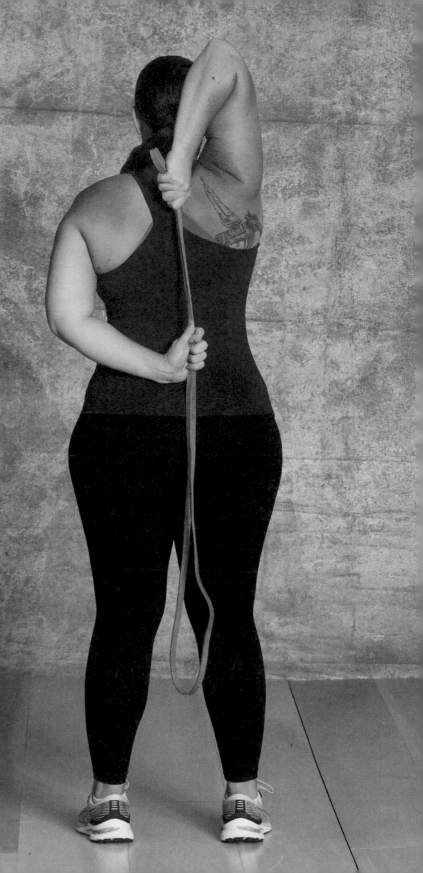

| LEVEL 1 | LEVEL 2 | LEVEL 3 | LEVEL 4 |

SHOULDER FLOSSING

SETUP Stand with feet hip-width apart. Dangle a band behind your neck with one hand, elbow bent and pointed toward the ceiling, then reach around your low back with the other hand to grab the band near your lower back.

STEP 1 Inhale and gently pull the band with your upper hand.

STEP 2 Exhale and gently pull the band with your lower hand. Continue alternating to "floss" your shoulders for the prescribed amount of time then repeat on the opposite side.

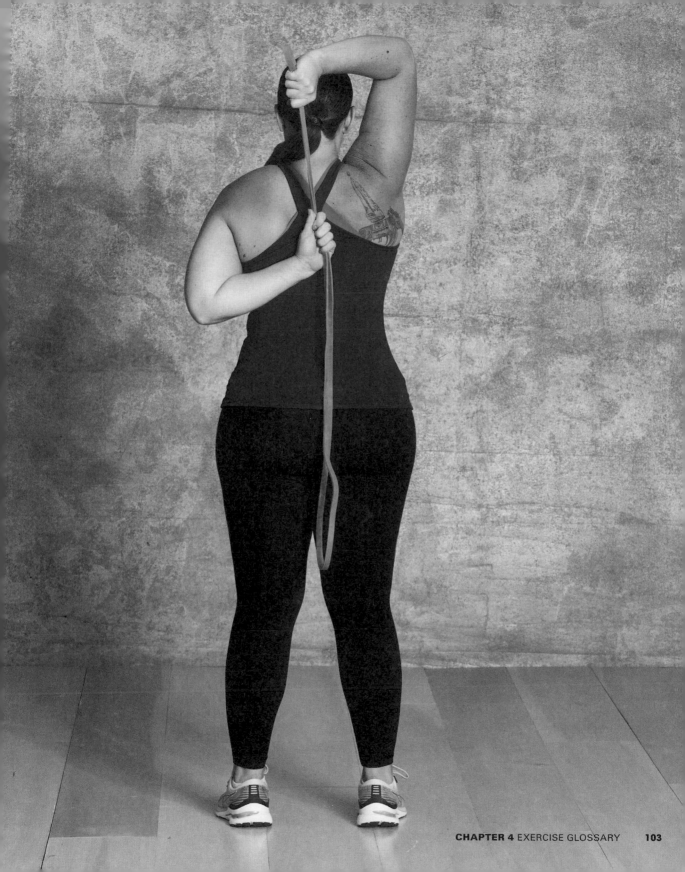

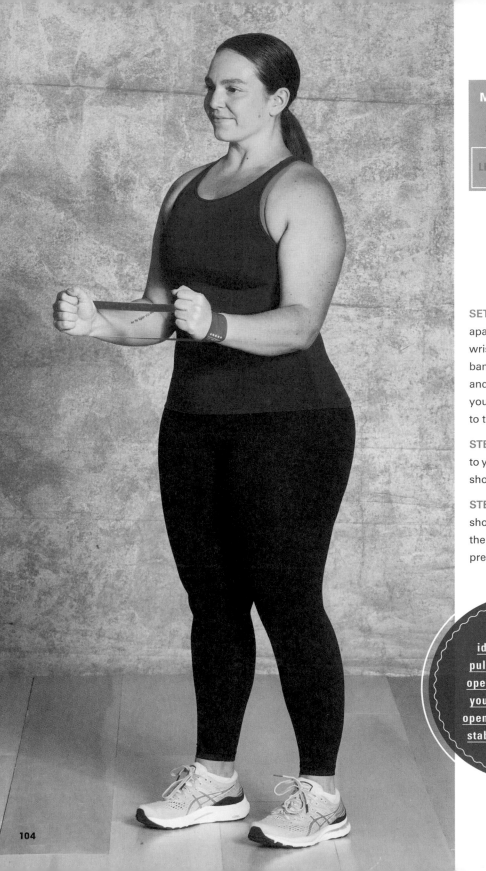

ISOMETRIC "W" HOLDS AT 90 DEGREES

SETUP Stand with feet hip-width apart, a mini loop around your wrists or holding one end of a long band in each hand, hands facing in and clenched. Glue your elbows to your sides, your forearms parallel to the ground.

STEP 1 Keeping your elbows glued to your sides, inhale and anchor your shoulders down toward your hips.

STEP 2 Exhale, squeezing your shoulder blades together as you pull the band apart. Hold for the prescribed amount of time.

This is identical to "W" pulls but instead of opening and closing your arms, hold the open position to build stability endurance.

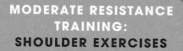

LEVEL 1	LEVEL 2	LEVEL 3	LEVEL 4

ISOMETRIC VERTICAL ABDUCTIONS

SETUP Stand with feet hip-width apart, arms straight overhead with a mini loop around your wrists or holding one end of a long band in each hand, palms facing out.

STEP 1 Inhale to anchor your shoulders down toward your hips.

STEP 2 Exhale, pulling the band apart while focusing on pinching your sides with your shoulder blades. Hold for the prescribed amount of time.

Use short tension-filled breaths as you hold the final position. Our deepest core muscles are the pelvic floor and diaphragm, so how you breathe will affect your core stability during movement. In exercises like this we want to keep tension through both our inhales and exhales to keep the core in its role as stabilizer.

Moderate Resistance Training

Push Exercises

Push-ups are one of the most popular pushing exercises there is—and for some, the most dreaded. But it doesn't have to be that way. This series of exercises can get you to a full push-up without ever getting on the ground. Plus, you'll strengthen your pec muscles, which along with your other posture muscles help support your breast tissue. If you have a larger bust, training these muscles is really nonnegotiable. A larger bust means you carry more weight higher up on your body, forcing your core and posture muscles to work harder to keep you upright. Strengthen those muscles and you'll protect your posture plus ward off back aches. You'll want to focus your attention on a few major areas during these exercises. As you lower your chest in these moves, think about your mid-back muscles that cradle under your shoulders and the area between your shoulder blades. As you raise yourself back up, you want to feel your core lift and your chest muscles or pecs and biceps push the wall or chair away.

AT A GLANCE

**Level 1:
Wall Scaptions**
p.107

**Level 2:
Elevated Banded
Push-Ups**
p.108

**Level 3:
Decrease
Elevation Banded
Push-Ups** p.109

**Level 4:
Elevated Banded
Back Push-Ups**
p.110

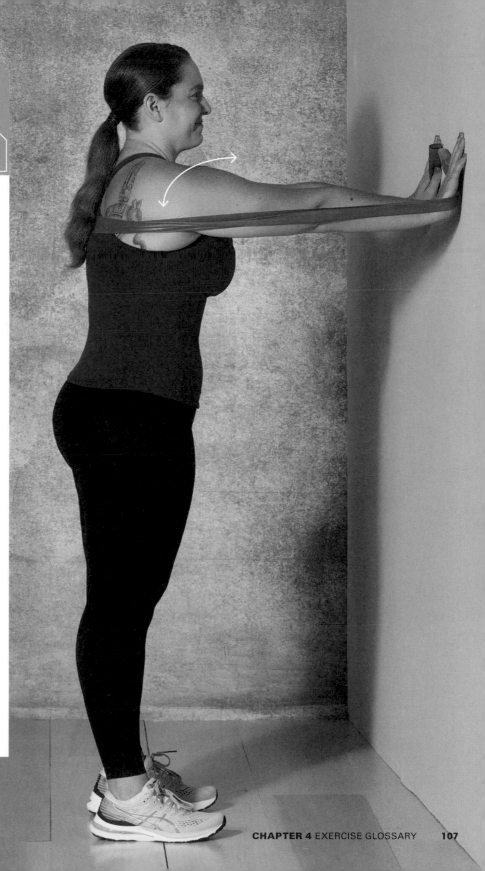

WALL SCAPTIONS

SETUP Stand arm's-length in front of a wall with feet hip-width apart and a long loop or long band around your back and arms, one end in each hand. Place your hands on the wall about shoulder-width apart, fingers spread as wide as possible. Lean slightly into the wall, pushing a little more into your fingers.

STEP 1 Anchor your shoulders down toward your hips, keeping them low and straight. Try to push the wall away creating a very slight doming sensation between your shoulder blades.

STEP 2 Try to pull your sternum to the wall while keeping your arms straight, aiming to kiss the bottom of your shoulder blades together behind you. Return to the starting position. Continue for the prescribed amount of time.

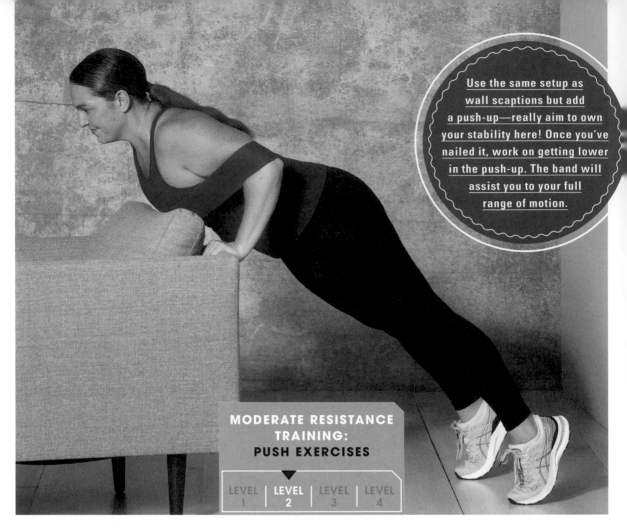

Use the same setup as wall scaptions but add a push-up—really aim to own your stability here! Once you've nailed it, work on getting lower in the push-up. The band will assist you to your full range of motion.

MODERATE RESISTANCE TRAINING:
PUSH EXERCISES

LEVEL 1 | LEVEL 2 | LEVEL 3 | LEVEL 4

ELEVATED BANDED PUSH-UPS

SETUP Stand arm's-length behind an armchair or couch with feet hip-width apart and a mini loop around your arms just above your elbows. Place your hands on the back of the chair about shoulder-width apart, fingers spread as wide as possible. Lean slightly into the chair, pushing a little more into your fingers.

STEP 1 Anchor your shoulders down toward your hips, with straight arms and a slight doming sensation.

STEP 2 Bend your elbows, as if you're trying to pull the chair to you.

STEP 3 Return to the starting position, straightening your arms as if you could push the chair through the floor. Continue for the prescribed amount of time.

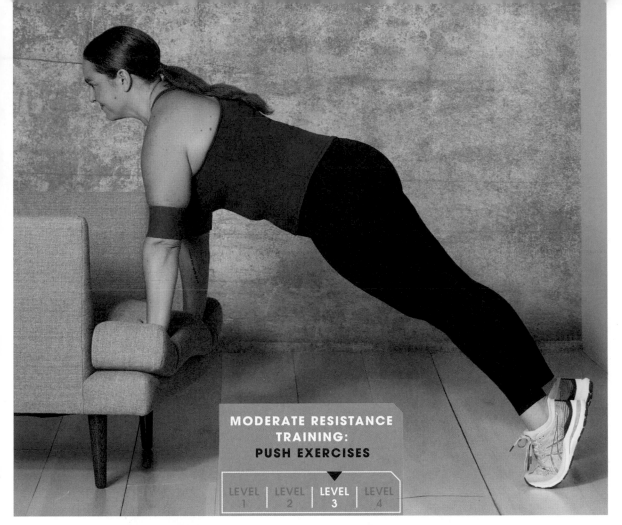

DECREASE ELEVATION BANDED PUSH-UPS

SETUP Assume a push-up position with a mini loop around your arms just above your elbows and your hands on the seat of an armchair. Place your hands shoulder-width apart, fingers spread as wide as possible.

STEP 1 Anchor your shoulders down toward your hips, with straight arms and a slight doming sensation.

STEP 2 Bend your elbows, as if you're trying to pull the chair to you.

STEP 3 Return to the starting position, straightening your arms as if you could push the chair through the floor. Continue for the prescribed amount of time.

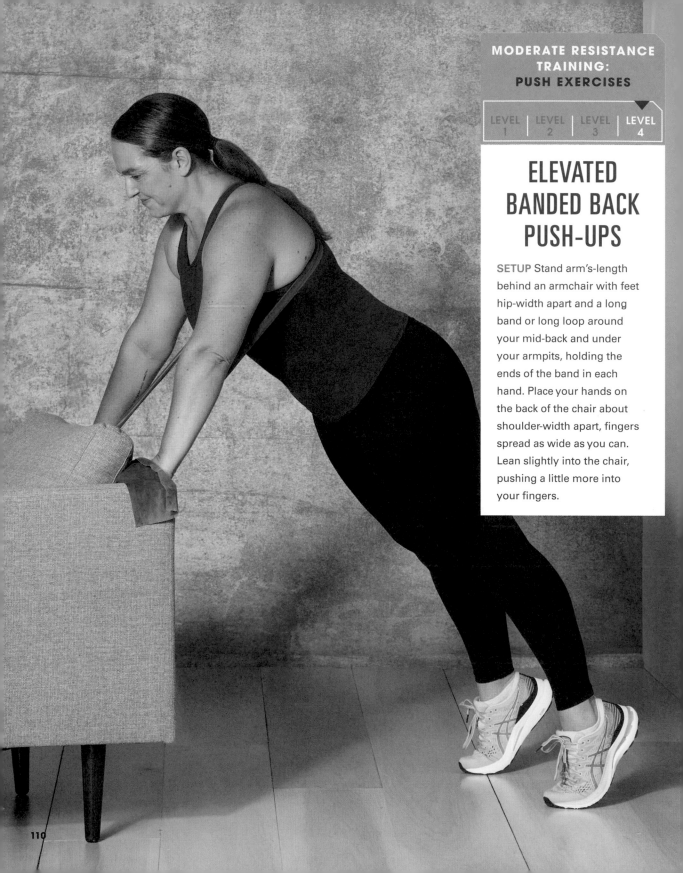

LEVEL 1	LEVEL 2	LEVEL 3	LEVEL 4

ELEVATED BANDED BACK PUSH-UPS

SETUP Stand arm's-length behind an armchair with feet hip-width apart and a long band or long loop around your mid-back and under your armpits, holding the ends of the band in each hand. Place your hands on the back of the chair about shoulder-width apart, fingers spread as wide as you can. Lean slightly into the chair, pushing a little more into your fingers.

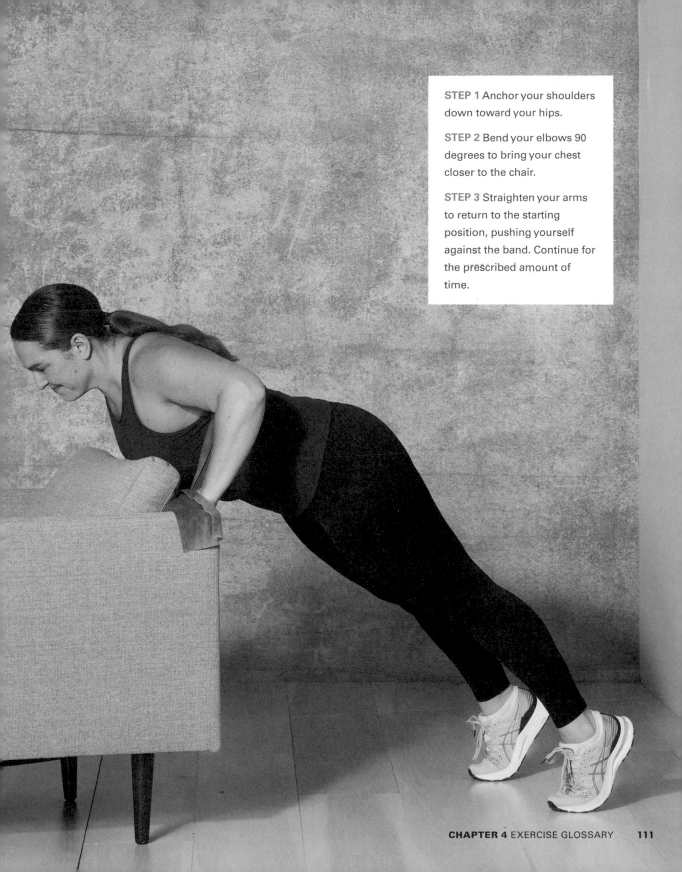

STEP 1 Anchor your shoulders down toward your hips.

STEP 2 Bend your elbows 90 degrees to bring your chest closer to the chair.

STEP 3 Straighten your arms to return to the starting position, pushing yourself against the band. Continue for the prescribed amount of time.

Moderate Resistance Training

Pull Exercises

If you ever felt like you needed a good stretch after sitting all day (who hasn't?), you'll love this series of posture-correcting exercises. They help loosen chronic tightness in your upper body, which can trigger everything from headaches and migraines to difficulty concentrating, heartburn, and even conditions like anxiety and depression. This series builds upon the pull-aparts you learned in the Light Resistance Training workout. You'll get the same arm-strengthening benefits, now with an added upper-body stretch as you work your way to the final exercise in this progression, bilateral around the worlds. For all these moves, you still want to feel those mid-back muscles that cradle underneath and in between the shoulder blades but you also want to feel a connection from those muscles to your triceps, or the back of your arms.

AT A GLANCE

**Level 1:
Pull-Aparts**
p.113

**Level 2:
Pull-Aparts
Low/High**
p.114

**Level 3:
Single-Arm
Around the
Worlds** p.116

**Level 4:
Bilateral Around
the Worlds**
p.117

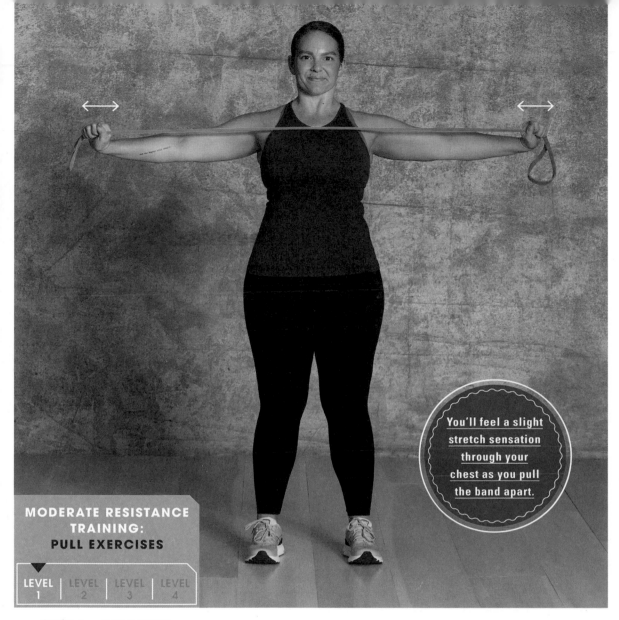

MODERATE RESISTANCE TRAINING: PULL EXERCISES

| LEVEL 1 | LEVEL 2 | LEVEL 3 | LEVEL 4 |

PULL-APARTS

SETUP Stand with feet hip-width apart, arms extended shoulder-width apart in front of you holding one end of a long band in each hand, palms facing out.

STEP 1 Inhale to anchor shoulder blades down toward your hips.

STEP 2 Exhale and squeeze your shoulder blades together, pulling the band apart with a slight bend in your elbows.

STEP 3 Return to the starting position. Continue for the prescribed amount of time.

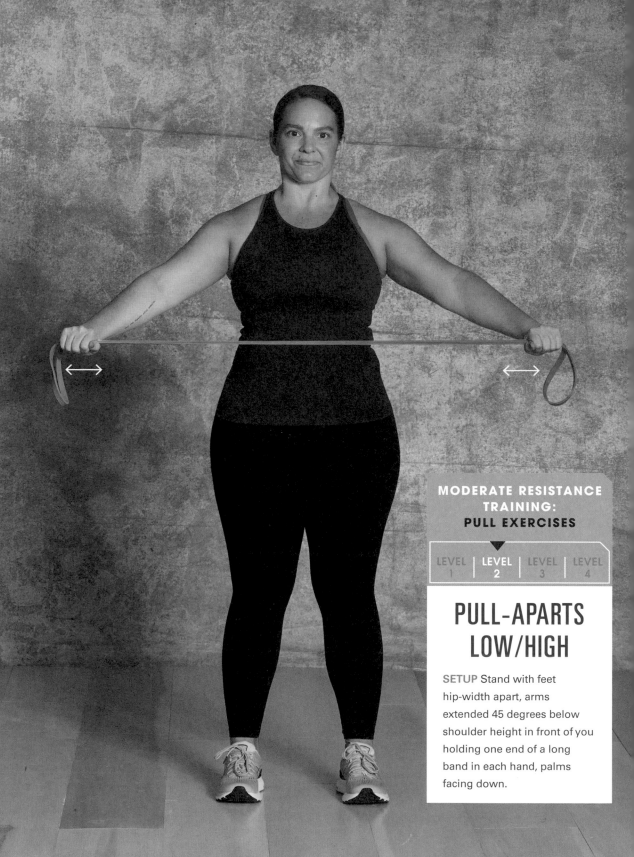

LEVEL 1	LEVEL 2	LEVEL 3	LEVEL 4

PULL-APARTS LOW/HIGH

SETUP Stand with feet hip-width apart, arms extended 45 degrees below shoulder height in front of you holding one end of a long band in each hand, palms facing down.

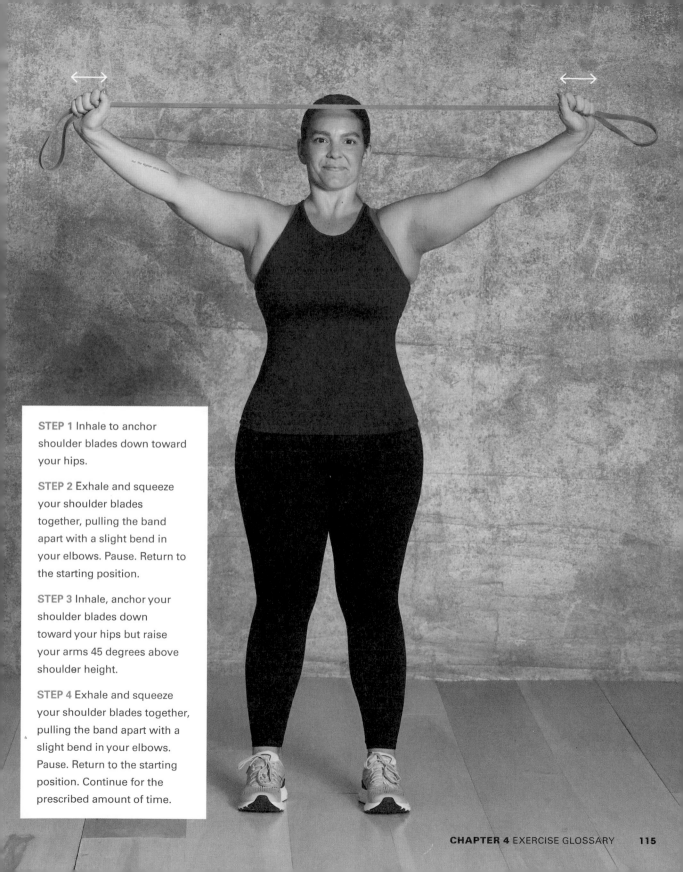

STEP 1 Inhale to anchor shoulder blades down toward your hips.

STEP 2 Exhale and squeeze your shoulder blades together, pulling the band apart with a slight bend in your elbows. Pause. Return to the starting position.

STEP 3 Inhale, anchor your shoulder blades down toward your hips but raise your arms 45 degrees above shoulder height.

STEP 4 Exhale and squeeze your shoulder blades together, pulling the band apart with a slight bend in your elbows. Pause. Return to the starting position. Continue for the prescribed amount of time.

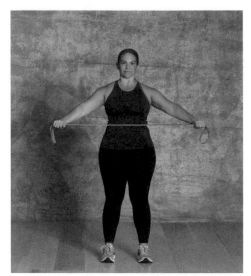

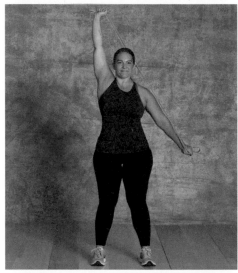

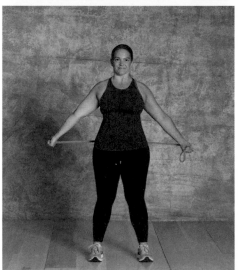

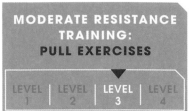

| LEVEL 1 | LEVEL 2 | LEVEL 3 | LEVEL 4 |

SINGLE-ARM AROUND THE WORLDS

SETUP Stand with feet hip-width apart while holding one end of a long band in each hand, arms straight down and slightly wider than your thighs.

STEP 1 Anchor your left hand at your side.

STEP 2 Reach your right hand forward, up, back, and down behind your back to tap the band on your glute then reverse the motion to return to your starting position. Continue for the prescribed amount of time then repeat on the opposite side.

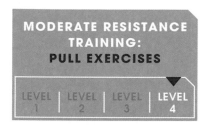

BILATERAL AROUND THE WORLDS

SETUP Stand with feet hip-width apart while holding one end of a long band in each hand, arms straight down.

STEP 1 Pull the band apart so your right hand is slightly to the right of your right thigh and your left hand is slightly to the left of your left thigh.

STEP 2 Reach both hands forward, up, back, and down behind your back to tap the band on your glutes then reverse the motion to return to your starting position. Continue for the prescribed amount of time.

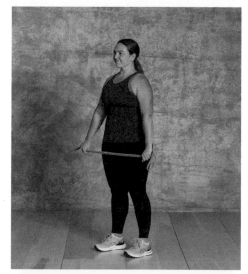

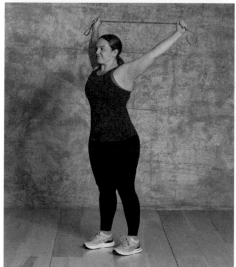

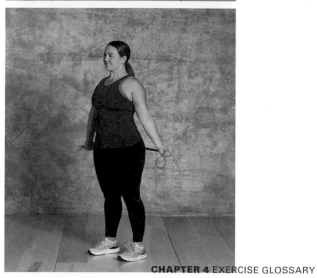

Moderate Resistance Training

Hip Hinge Exercises

Improving your hip hinge will help you achieve almost any fitness goal you might have. As you discovered on page 86, a solid hip hinge makes daily tasks like bending down to tie your shoes easier. The work you did in the Light Resistance Training hip hinge series helps you build the foundation for moves like those in this series, which will torch your legs and tone your lower body. These exercises are all about the backs of your thighs (a.k.a. your hamstrings) working together with the glutes. So when hinging back you want to feel a stretching sensation in your hamstrings. To return back up, think about pushing the floor away and squeezing your glutes forward.

AT A GLANCE

Level 1:
Good Mornings
p.119

Level 2:
RDLs
p.120

Level 3:
Single-Leg RDLs
p.122

Level 4:
Deadlifts
p.123

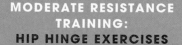

| LEVEL 1 | LEVEL 2 | LEVEL 3 | LEVEL 4 |

GOOD MORNINGS

SETUP Stand facing away from a wall or back of a couch (about a foot's-length away), feet hip-width apart. Wrap a long band around your back near the base of your shoulder blades and around your arms, pulling the ends to reach your hands straight in front of you.

STEP 1 Inhale, pulling the band forward as you hinge your hips to lightly tap the wall behind you. Try to keep your weight in the center of your feet or even slightly forward into your spread-out toes, only to the point where you can keep your heels down.

STEP 2 Return to the starting position. Continue for the prescribed amount of time.

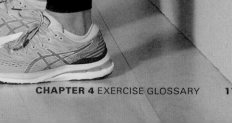

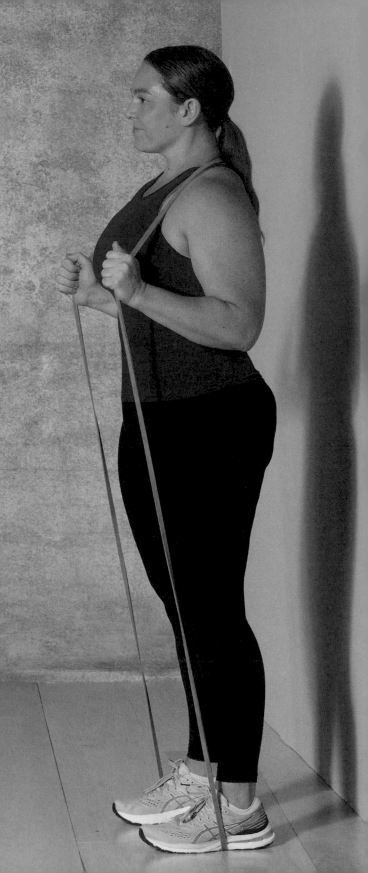

| LEVEL 1 | LEVEL 2 | LEVEL 3 | LEVEL 4 |

RDLS

SETUP Stand facing away from a wall or back of a couch (about a foot's-length away), feet hip-width apart. Loop a long loop under the arches of your feet, wrapping the top of the loop around your shoulders and grabbing the band at chest level.

STEP 1 Inhale, hinging your hips to lightly tap the wall behind you. Try to keep your weight in the center of your feet or even slightly forward into your spread-out toes, only to the point where you can keep your heels down.

STEP 2 Return to the starting position. Continue for the prescribed amount of time.

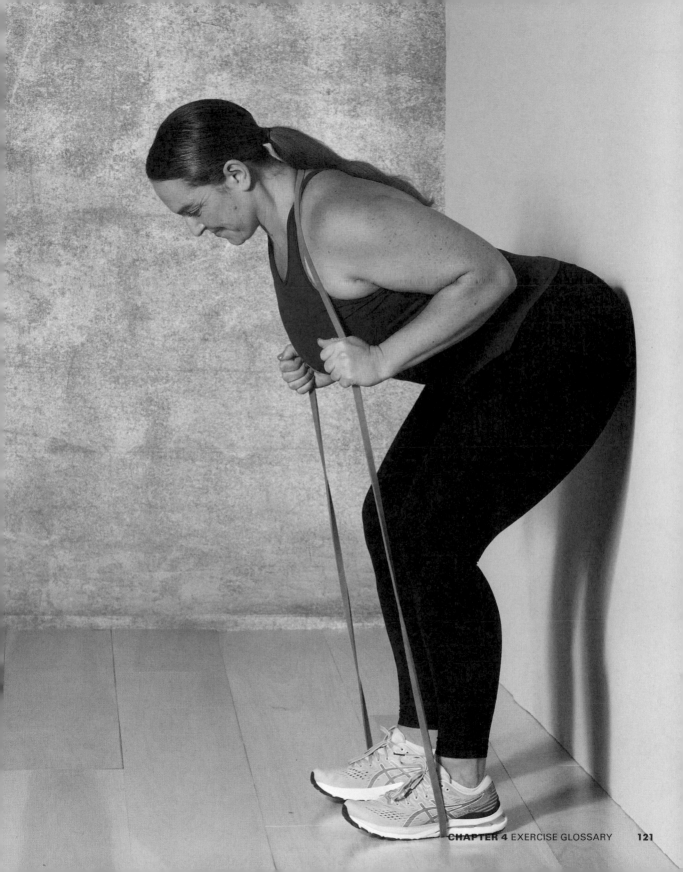

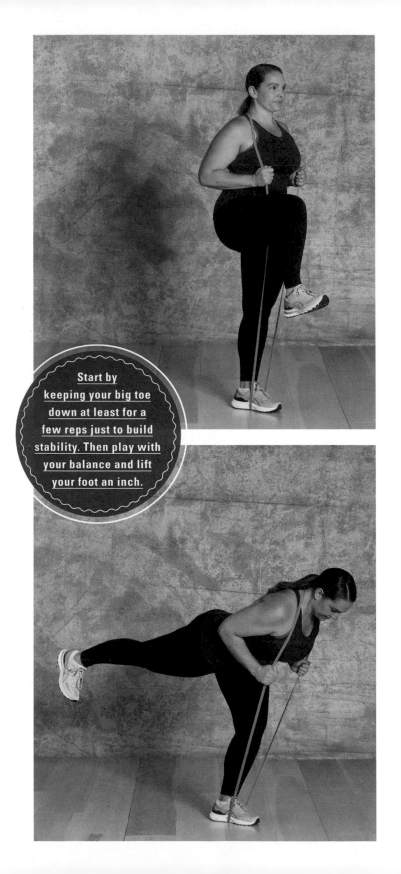

Start by keeping your big toe down at least for a few reps just to build stability. Then play with your balance and lift your foot an inch.

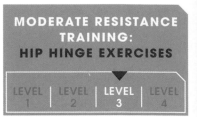
SINGLE-LEG RDLS

SETUP Stand with feet hip-width apart, a long band over your shoulders and looped under the arch of your left foot. Grip the band at waist level and raise your right thigh so it's parallel to the floor.

STEP 1 Inhale, hinging your hips back while shifting your head, chest, and hips over the center of your left foot. Extend your right leg back as you hinge. Squeeze your glutes to prevent your hips from moving with your leg.

STEP 2 Return to the starting position. Continue for for the prescribed amount of time then repeat on the opposite side.

LEVEL 1	LEVEL 2	LEVEL 3	LEVEL 4

DEADLIFTS

SETUP Stand with feet hip-width apart with a long band under both feet and holding the ends in each hand, arms at your sides.

STEP 1 Inhale, hinging your hips back and keeping your proud chest over your feet to feel a big stretch in your hamstrings. Keeping your arms straight, pull as much slack out of the band as you can.

STEP 2 Exhale and return to standing by squeezing your glutes forward to push yourself like opening a book. Continue for the prescribed amount of time.

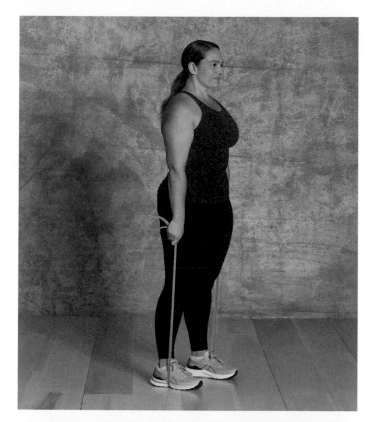

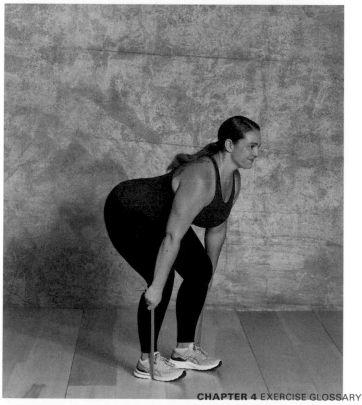

Moderate Resistance Training

Single-Leg Exercises

To strengthen your lower body and core, you don't need to amp up the effort to 11. These exercises require just a little more intensity than the standing kickbacks you do in your Light Resistance Training, but deliver even greater toning results. The difference? Bending your legs. In each of these moves you'll bring one of your legs closer to your chest, either by lifting it (as you will in marching and bird dogs) or by bending it (as in step-ups and split squats). Movements like this activate both your core and your legs. Your core works to flex your hip and your hamstring works to stabilize your body. During the marching and bird dog exercises you can focus on using your core to move the legs. On the step-up and split squat, focus on connecting that same core pressure to the front leg.

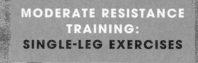

| LEVEL 1 | LEVEL 2 | LEVEL 3 | LEVEL 4 |

MARCHING

SETUP Stand with feet hip-width apart, a band around your arches.

STEP 1 Inhale to shift your head, chest, and hips over your left foot.

STEP 2 Exhale to slowly lift your right knee up, aiming to raise it parallel to the ground by the end of your exhale.

STEP 3 Inhale to return to the starting position. Repeat on the opposite side. Continue alternating sides for the prescribed amount of time.

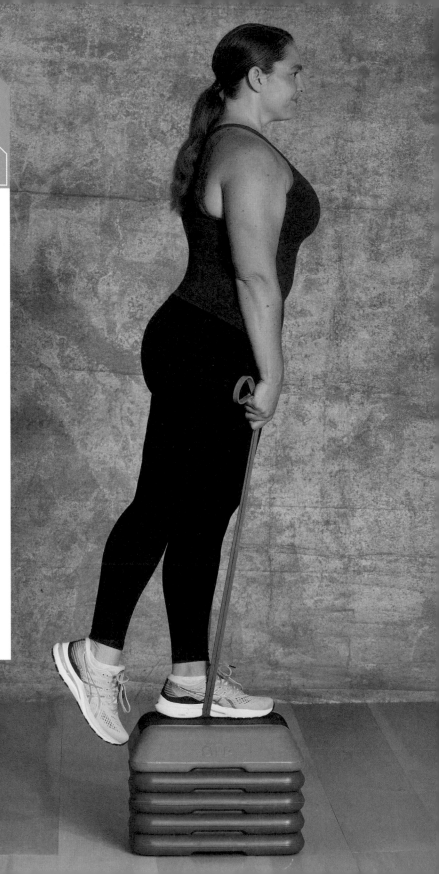

STEP-UPS

SETUP Stand with feet hip-width apart facing a set of stairs or a box that can support your weight. Place your left foot on a long band on the first step (preferably with your whole foot but as long as your foot feels stable it'll work). Hold the ends of the band in each hand.

STEP 1 Inhale, shifting forward so most of your weight is over your left foot.

STEP 2 Exhale, raise yourself up to a straight leg, driving down through your left foot.

STEP 3 Step back down, bringing your left foot in line with your right. Continue for the prescribed amount of time then repeat on the opposite side.

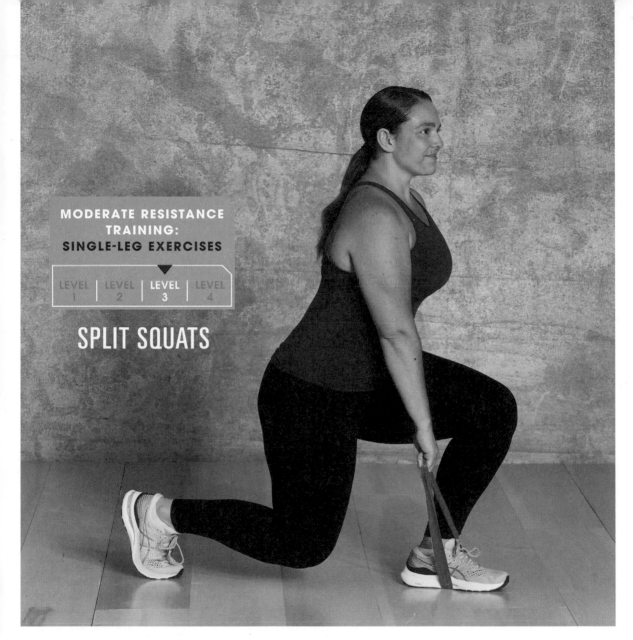

| LEVEL 1 | LEVEL 2 | **LEVEL 3** | LEVEL 4 |

SPLIT SQUATS

SETUP Stand with feet slightly wider than hip-width apart, a long band under your left foot, the end in your right hand. Slide your right foot straight back about two foot-lengths behind you, leading with your heel. Allow your right heel to lift and gently push outward.

STEP 1 Inhale and sit your hips straight down, trying to keep your weight even between your front and back foot. Make your chest slightly more proud as you sit.

STEP 2 Exhale, raising yourself back to standing by pushing down through both feet. Pull your right glute forward slightly to keep your hips square. Continue for the prescribed amount of time then repeat on the opposite side.

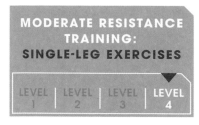

BIRD DOGS

SETUP Stand slightly less than arm's-length from a wall or back of an armchair, hands on the back of the chair, feet hip-width apart. Place one end of a long loop under the arch of your left foot, holding the other end in your left hand.

STEP 1 Shift your head, chest, and hips over your right foot, raising your left foot slightly. Hinge into your hips and feel a slight stretching sensation in your left glute.

STEP 2 Inhale, anchoring your shoulder blades down.

STEP 3 Exhale, raising your left hand overhead and extending your left leg behind you, leading with your heel.

STEP 4 Inhale to control the return to the starting position. Continue for the prescribed amount of time then repeat on the opposite side.

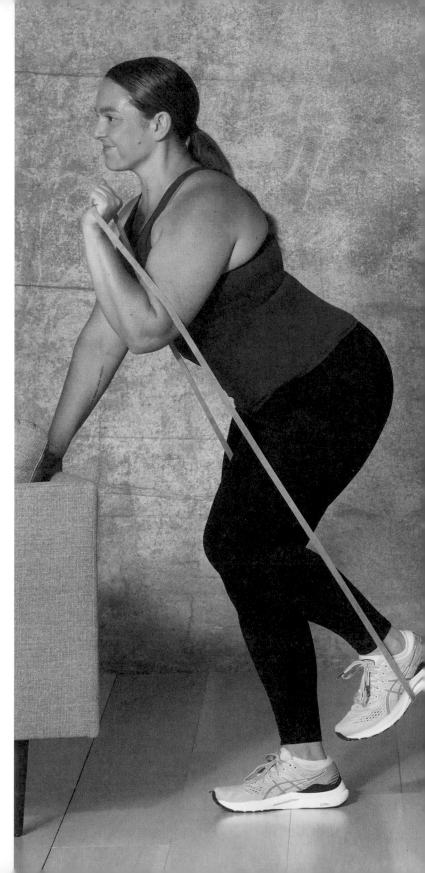

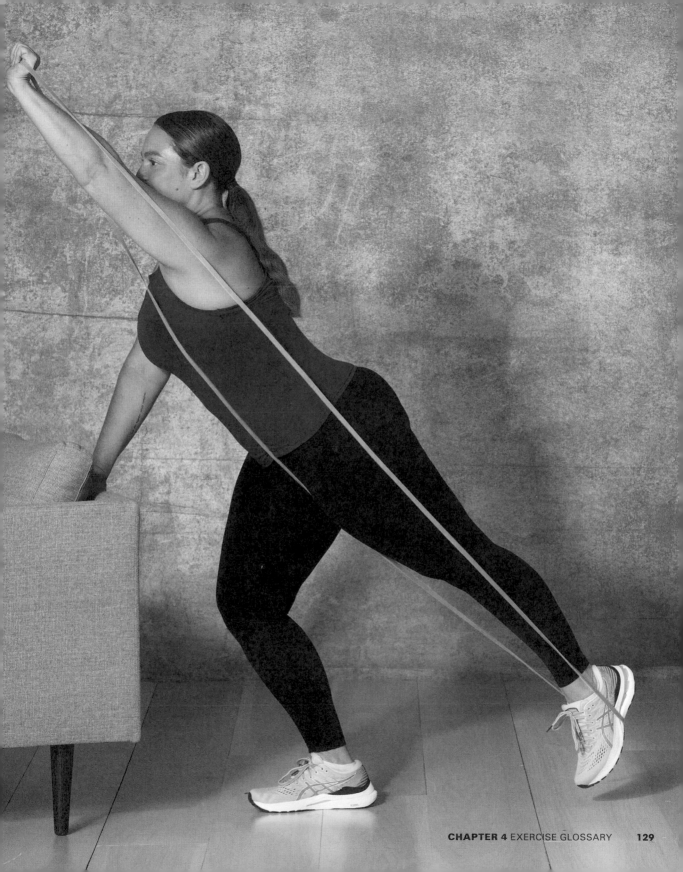

Moderate Resistance Training

Core Exercises

Here's some good news: You only need to learn one core exercise for your Moderate Resistance Training to fire up your midsection. That's because this particular move—chops—does so much with one simple motion. You'll strengthen the sides of your abs, or obliques, work your shoulders, and build core strength that will help you hoist up grocery bags or twist to grab your purse from the backseat with ease. Although the motion is uncomplicated, it can be challenging, so start slow the first week. If you're feeling strong by Week 3 or 4 you can try picking up your pace, which will add a bit of cardio to the move. It's especially important to take your time building this movement pattern if you're postpartum, experiencing low back tightness or digestive issues, or if you participate in sports or physical activities. This exercise is mostly about the obliques so that's definitely where you want to feel the work coming from. Your point of stability is actually both the hips and the shoulder girdle. Think about moving from those waist muscles but also add some tension to your glutes and mid-back muscles to generate stability, which will ensure you don't twist from your low back.

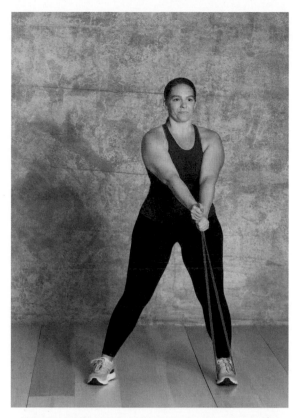

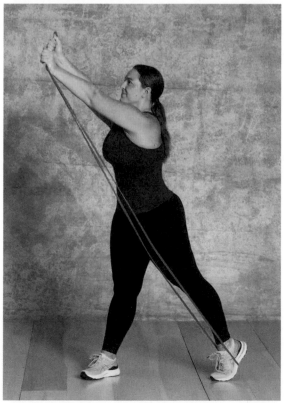

CHOPS

SETUP Stand with feet slightly wider than hip-width apart. Place a long loop under your left foot, holding the ends of the band in both hands, arms extended over your left leg about 45 degrees below shoulder level. Adjust the grip of the band to focus on the top or bottom ranges as you go along.

STEP 1 Inhale to reach your chest toward your left foot, sitting your hips back and bending your knees slightly.

STEP 2 Exhale and pull the band up diagonally toward the outside of your right shoulder like you're hitting a home run. Focus on pushing with your left hip as you pull the band diagonally upward, forcefully exhaling to get the most core engagement.

STEP 3 Return your chest back over your left foot. Continue for the prescribed amount of time then repeat on the opposite side.

All Out Resistance Training

Shoulder Exercises

For your final shoulder series, we'll use bands and gravity to challenge your shoulders and build more strength. You'll get even more of the good stuff that our other shoulder series offer: pain-free movement, a greater range of motion, and toned muscles. Together, that means greater weight loss success and better movement for life. For this series you should feel your mid-back muscles working but also the smaller shoulder muscles like the rotator cuff and deltoids, both of which are right by your shoulder joints.

AT A GLANCE

Level 1: Isometric Shoulder Abductions p.133

Level 2: Banded Hand Taps p.134

Level 3: Shoulder Circles p.135

Level 4: Vertical Shoulder Circles p.136

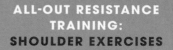
ISOMETRIC SHOULDER ABDUCTIONS

SETUP Stand with feet hip-width apart. Anchor one end of the band either by tying it to a doorknob or looping it under the arch of your right foot. Hold the other end in your right hand, arm down at your side.

STEP 1 Inhale, anchoring your shoulder blades down toward your hips.

STEP 2 Exhale, pulling your right arm out to the side keeping your shoulder down and chest proud.

STEP 3 Return to the starting position. Continue for the prescribed amount of time then repeat on the opposite side.

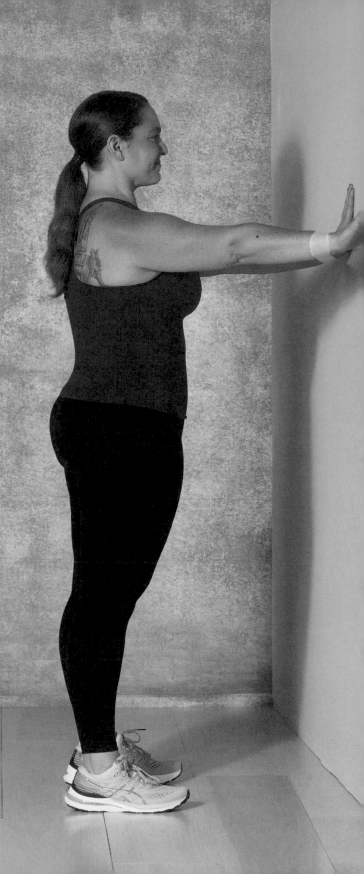

| LEVEL 1 | LEVEL 2 | LEVEL 3 | LEVEL 4 |

BANDED HAND TAPS

SETUP Stand arm's-length in front of a wall with feet hip-width apart and a mini loop around your wrists. Place your hands on the wall about shoulder-width apart.

STEP 1 Shift your weight to your left hand while simultaneously sliding your right hand four inches or so to the right. Try not to sink into your left shoulder. Using short tension-filled breaths, continuously aim to push the wall away with your left hand.

STEP 2 Slide your right hand back to the starting position. Continue for the prescribed amount of time then repeat on the opposite side.

To make this move more challenging, try it on the ground in plank position.

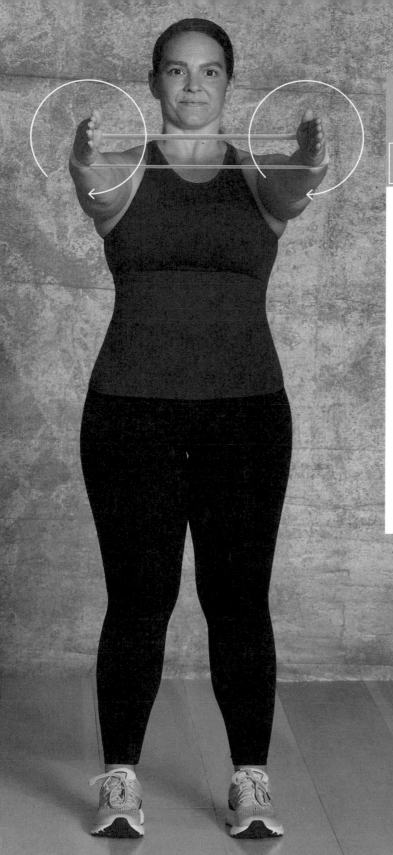

LEVEL 1	LEVEL 2	LEVEL 3	LEVEL 4

SHOULDER CIRCLES

SETUP Stand with feet hip-width apart and a mini loop around your wrists. Lift your arms in front of you to shoulder height.

STEP 1 Make a small, controlled clockwise circle with your hands, then reverse it, maintaining tension in the loop. Use short, tension-filled breaths and anchor your shoulders down. Continue for the prescribed amount of time.

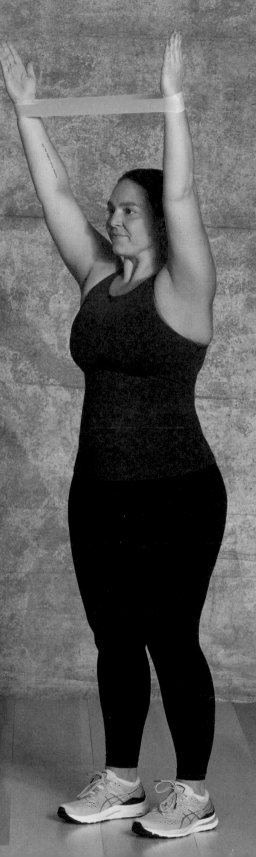

LEVEL 1	LEVEL 2	LEVEL 3	LEVEL 4

VERTICAL SHOULDER CIRCLES

SETUP Stand with feet hip-width apart and a mini loop around your wrists. Raise your arms straight over your head, aiming to line your biceps up by your ears with your shoulder blades anchoring toward your hips.

STEP 1 Using short, tension-filled breaths, make small circles outward with your arms, then reverse it, maintaining tension in the loop. Continue for the prescribed amount of time.

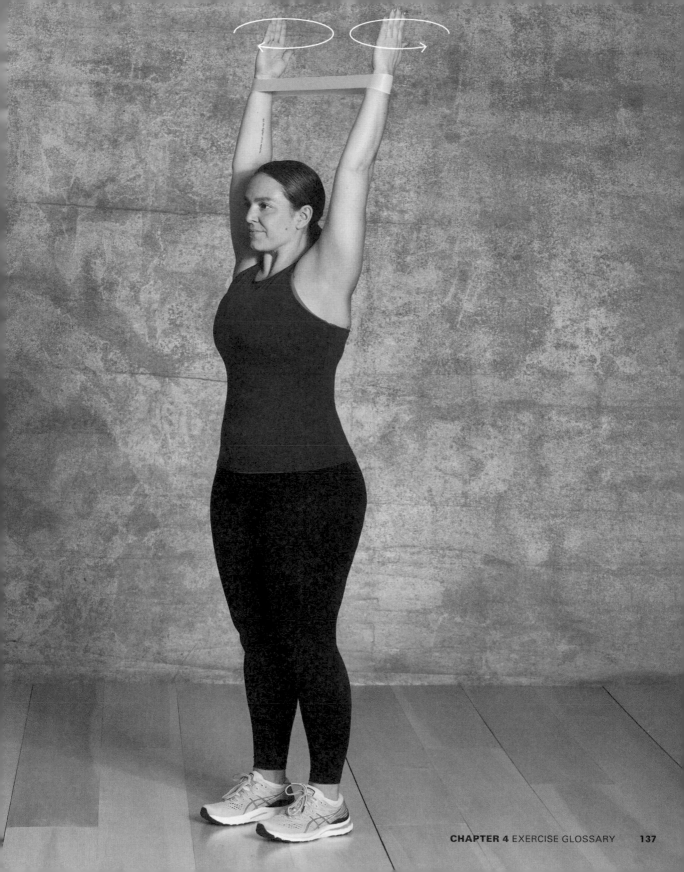

All Out Resistance Training

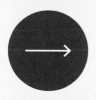

Push Exercises

So many of the benefits you get from push-ups can be achieved without cranking out dozens of sets. Our final series of push exercises isolates many of the key motions used in a push-up but adapts them so they can be done standing up or leaning against an armchair or wall. The result is stronger, more toned arms with less pressure on your joints. Not sure if you're doing it right? You should feel these moves in your mid-back, pecs, and biceps as you push your arms.

AT A GLANCE

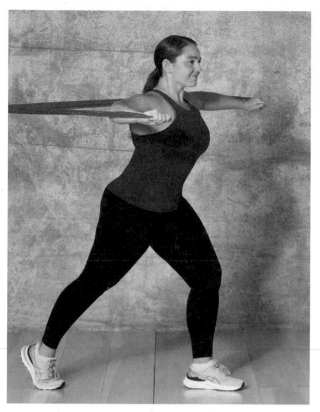

CHEST FLYS

SETUP Anchor a long band to a doorknob. Facing away from the doorknob, grip the band in each hand. Extend your arms in front of you with a slight bend as if you were hugging a big beach ball. Step your right foot back so your feet are staggered.

STEP 1 Inhale and open your arms like you're hugging a larger beach ball, squeezing your shoulder blades together behind you.

STEP 2 Exhale and hug your arms back around your smaller beach ball, keeping your chest proud. Continue for the prescribed amount of time.

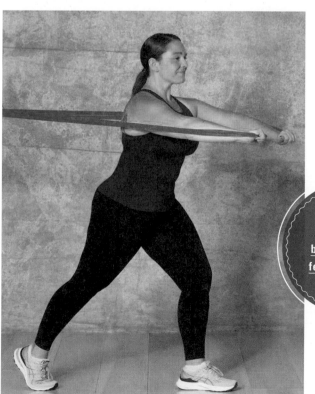

Adjust your grip on the band until you feel your chest engage.

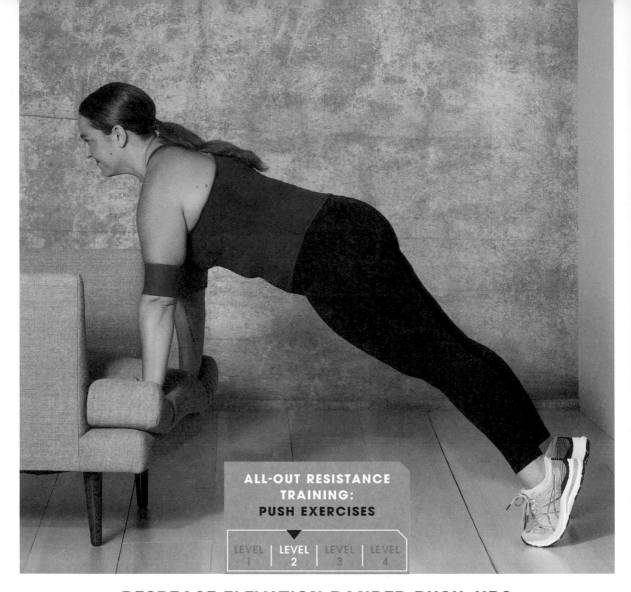

ALL-OUT RESISTANCE
TRAINING:
PUSH EXERCISES

| LEVEL 1 | LEVEL 2 | LEVEL 3 | LEVEL 4 |

DECREASE ELEVATION BANDED PUSH-UPS

SETUP Assume a push-up position with a mini loop around your arms just above your elbows and your hands on the back of a couch or stable chair. Place your hands shoulder-width apart, fingers spread as wide as possible.

STEP 1 Anchor your shoulders down toward your hips, keeping them low and straight. Try to push the couch or chair away creating a very slight doming sensation between your shoulder blades.

STEP 2 Bend your elbows 90 degrees to bring your chest closer to the couch.

STEP 3 Straighten your arms to return to the starting position. Continue for the prescribed amount of time.

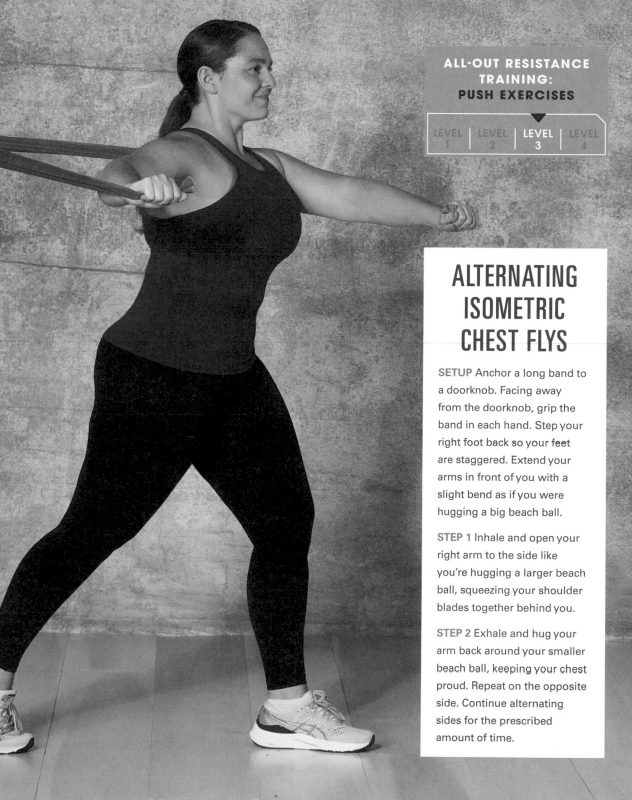

ALTERNATING ISOMETRIC CHEST FLYS

SETUP Anchor a long band to a doorknob. Facing away from the doorknob, grip the band in each hand. Step your right foot back so your feet are staggered. Extend your arms in front of you with a slight bend as if you were hugging a big beach ball.

STEP 1 Inhale and open your right arm to the side like you're hugging a larger beach ball, squeezing your shoulder blades together behind you.

STEP 2 Exhale and hug your arm back around your smaller beach ball, keeping your chest proud. Repeat on the opposite side. Continue alternating sides for the prescribed amount of time.

LEVEL 1	LEVEL 2	LEVEL 3	LEVEL 4

SINGLE-ARM VERTICAL PUSHES

SETUP Stand with feet hip-width apart. Place either the long loop or the long open band around the arch of your left foot, holding the other end in your left hand, palm facing forward and at shoulder level. If you have limited vertical range (see test on opposite page), step your left foot back enough so when you raise your left arm as high as possible, you create a vertical line from your left foot to your left hand.

STEP 1 Inhale, anchoring your shoulder blades toward your hips and aiming to keep the shoulder anchored and wrapped around your ribs.

STEP 2 Exhale and push upward to raise your arm as high as you can without sticking out your ribs or leaning back.

STEP 3 Lower your arm to return to the starting position. Continue for the prescribed amount of time then repeat on the opposite side.

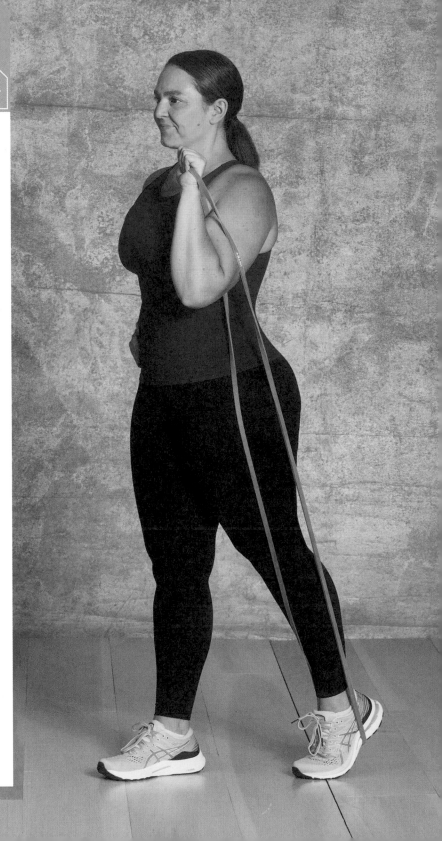

To nail your form, try this test to find your vertical range (or how high you can lift your arms).

- **Stand** with your heels, butt, ribs, and back of your head touching a wall.

- **Inhale**, anchoring your shoulder blades toward your hips.

- **Exhale**, raise your arms straight up until you either touch the wall or you lose one of your points of contact against the wall. This angle is where you start your overhead push journey.

All Out Resistance Training

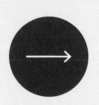

Pull Exercises

These moves give you double the bang for your buck. You'll tone your arms with pulling motions and fire up your glutes, hamstrings, and core thanks to the added hinge in the first three moves. You don't need to position your back parallel to the floor to work the right muscles here, so don't worry about getting all the way down. The one place you don't want to feel it? Your lower back. If you start to feel tension there, take a moment to pause and make sure you're in the correct position. If resetting doesn't quite fix it, try stabilizing your body by sitting a little further back into your hips and slightly lifting your chest until you feel your glutes pull the tension out of your back. You also want to feel those mid-back muscles, but one side at a time so also focus on keeping your nonworking side and hips stable.

AT A GLANCE

**Level 1:
Single-Arm
Bent-Over Rows**
p.145

**Level 2:
Bent-Over
Reverse Flys**
p.146

**Level 3:
Alternating
Single-Arm
Bent-Over Rows**
p.147

**Level 4:
Standing Vertical
Pull-Downs**
p.148

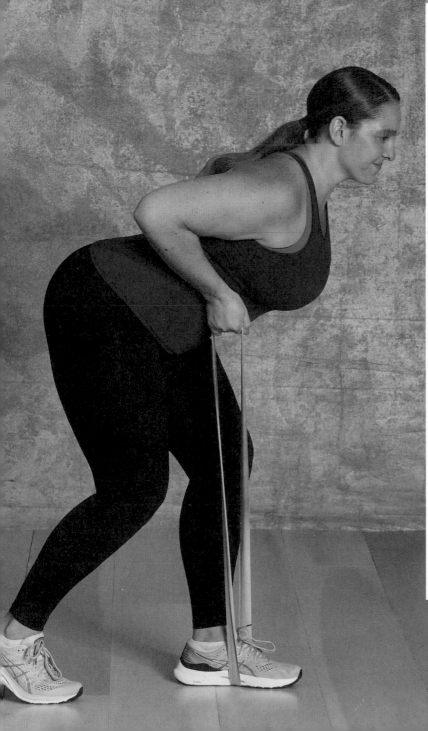

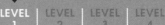

| LEVEL 1 | LEVEL 2 | LEVEL 3 | LEVEL 4 |

SINGLE-ARM BENT-OVER ROWS

SETUP Stand with feet hip-width apart, a mini loop around the arch of your left foot. Hold the end of the band in your right hand. Shift your head, chest, and hips over your left foot, tucking your right foot back slightly so just your toes are touching the floor, hips square. Hinge your hips back until your proud chest is about parallel to the floor, weight remaining over your left foot.

STEP 1 Inhale and pause for a moment. Then, exhale and raise your right hand to lightly tap your right ribs, driving your elbow straight up to the ceiling.

STEP 2 Inhale to straighten your arm and return to the starting position. Continue for the prescribed amount of time then repeat on the opposite side.

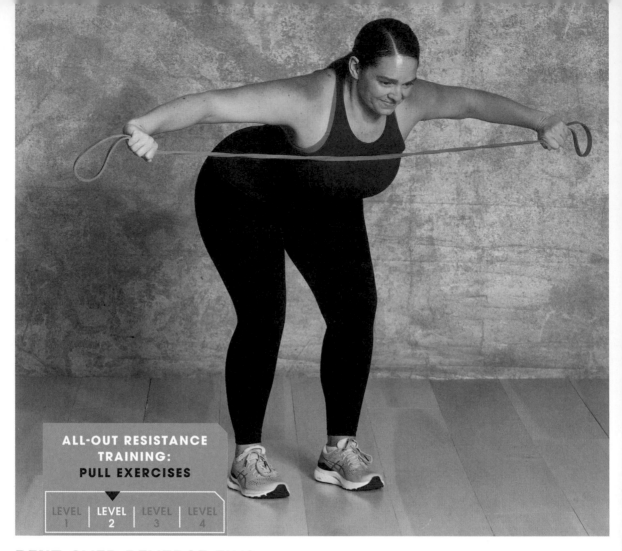

BENT-OVER REVERSE FLYS

SETUP Stand with your back about a foot's-length away from a wall or back of a couch, feet hip-width apart. With the long loop in your hands, hinge at the hips to lightly tap the wall behind your and to bring your proud spine as close to parallel to the floor, arms reaching for the floor.

STEP 1 Inhale, anchoring your shoulder blades down toward your hips.

STEP 2 Exhale, pulling your shoulder blades together while raising your arms out to your sides, keeping your arms straight.

STEP 3 Lower your arms to return to the starting position. Continue for the prescribed amount of time.

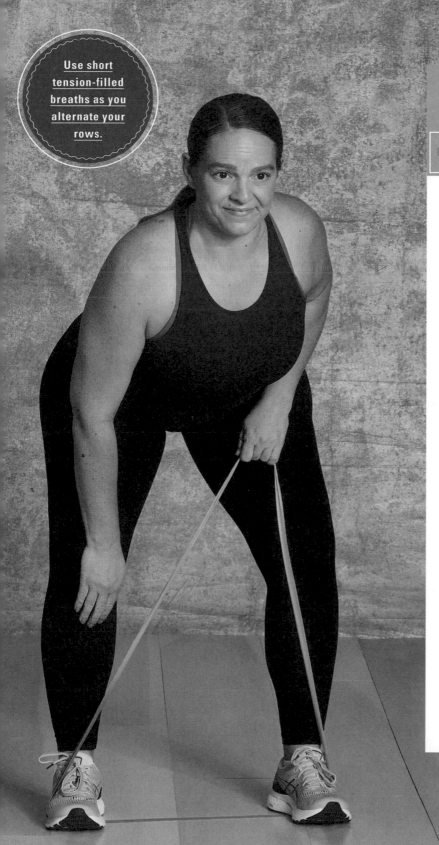

Use short tension-filled breaths as you alternate your rows.

ALL-OUT RESISTANCE TRAINING: PULL EXERCISES

| LEVEL 1 | LEVEL 2 | LEVEL 3 | LEVEL 4 |

ALTERNATING SINGLE-ARM BENT-OVER ROWS

SETUP Stand with feet hip-width apart, a mini loop around the arches of your feet. Hold the end of the band in your left hand. Hinge your hips back until your proud chest is about parallel to the floor.

STEP 1 Inhale, anchor your shoulder blades, and pause for a moment. Then, exhale to pull with your left hand and lightly tap your left hip bone, driving your elbow straight back to the ceiling.

STEP 2 Inhale to straighten your arm and return to the starting position. Grab the band with your right hand and repeat on your right side. Continue alternating sides for the prescribed amount of time.

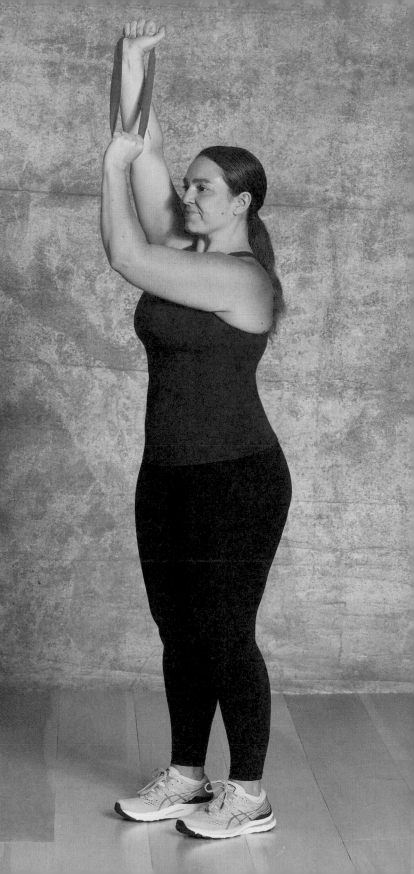

| LEVEL 1 | LEVEL 2 | LEVEL 3 | LEVEL 4 |

STANDING VERTICAL PULL-DOWNS

SETUP Stand with feet hip-width apart. (If you have limited vertical range, step your right foot back enough so when you raise your right arm as high as possible, you create a vertical line from your right foot to your right hand.) Place a mini loop on the palm of your right hand and raise it as high as possible. Grab the other end of the band with your left hand.

STEP 1 Inhale, anchoring both shoulder blades.

STEP 2 Exhale, pushing your right hand even higher as you pull your left hand down aiming your elbow for your waist and your hand for your armpit.

STEP 3 Return to the starting position. Continue for the prescribed amount of time then repeat on the opposite side.

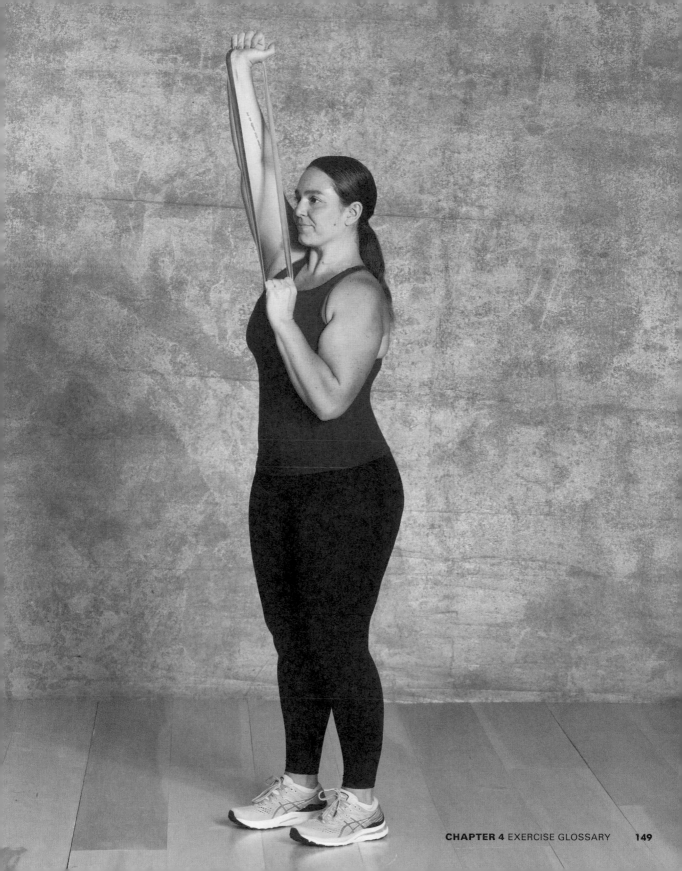

All Out Resistance Training

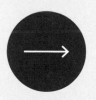

Hip Hinge Exercises

This series is all about squats, which are one of the most efficient exercises for toning your whole body. That's because you can easily layer other movements on top of them to increase your burn, like you'll do here. You'll add powerful moves like pull-aparts and heel raises, plus use bands to increase the resistance in this tried-and-true exercise.

To make sure you're getting the best burn possible, focus on a few key areas. On your way down, put your weight fully into both feet, not just the heels or balls of your feet. Your knees should reach over your middle toes. They can pull slightly toward your pinky toe on the way down and drive toward your big toe on the way up but not outside that lane. When you add the band around your legs, think about where your knees are pointing. Push your knees out slightly on the way down then pull them in slightly on the way up. This ensures you use the stabilizing muscles in your glutes, making them stronger and making you more stable and rooted in everything you do, from squats to running up stairs.

For the last exercise in this series, you'll layer in a heel raise to tone your calves, improve your balance, and even help alleviate plantar fasciitis pain. If you struggle standing on your toes, omit the pull-apart from this exercise and hold on to a wall for balance. The secret to a wobble-free lift is to think about raising your heel over the space between your big toe and second toe, while spreading your toes out. The more floor area your toes are in contact with, the easier it'll be to balance.

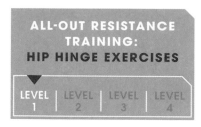

LEVEL 1 | LEVEL 2 | LEVEL 3 | LEVEL 4

SQUATS WITH PULL-APARTS

SETUP Stand with feet shoulder-width apart or a little wider, feet turned out slightly. Hold the ends of a long loop in your hands, palms facing down with arms stretched out in front of you.

STEP 1 Keeping your chest proud, inhale and bend your knees as you sink your hips like you're sitting in a chair, keeping your weight over your feet.

STEP 2 Exhale to return to standing, pulling the band apart with a slight bend in your elbows. Squeeze your shoulder blades together as you do.

STEP 3 Bring your arms back in front of you. Continue for the prescribed amount of time.

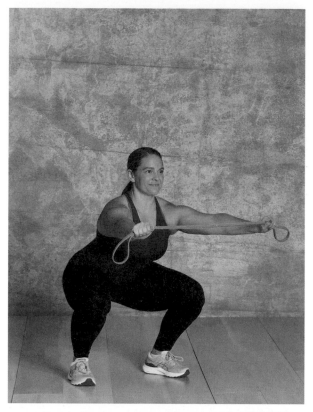

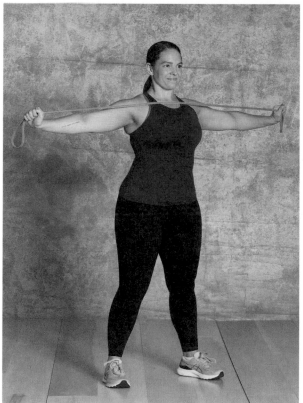

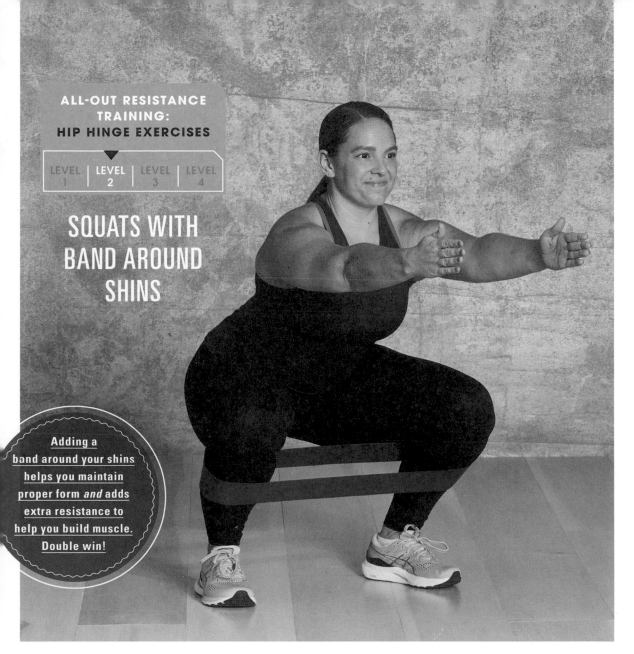

LEVEL 1	LEVEL 2	LEVEL 3	LEVEL 4

SQUATS WITH BAND AROUND SHINS

Adding a band around your shins helps you maintain proper form *and* adds extra resistance to help you build muscle. Double win!

SETUP Place a mini loop band around your shins about halfway up to your knees. Stand with feet shoulder-width apart or a little wider, feet turned out slightly, arms extended in front of you.

STEP 1 Keeping your chest proud, inhale to bend your knees as you sink your hips like you're sitting in a chair, keeping your weight over your feet. Maintain tension against the band to feel the outside of your glutes engage.

STEP 2 Exhale to push yourself back up controlling the tension in the band. Continue for the prescribed amount of time.

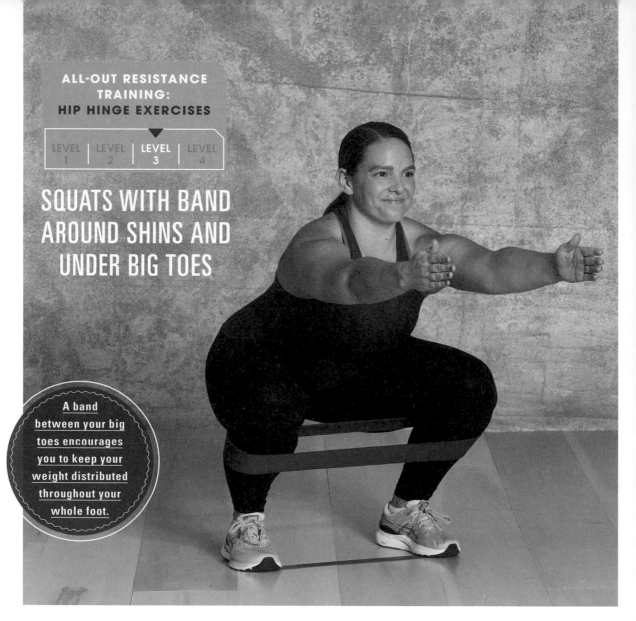

| LEVEL 1 | LEVEL 2 | LEVEL 3 | LEVEL 4 |

SQUATS WITH BAND AROUND SHINS AND UNDER BIG TOES

A band between your big toes encourages you to keep your weight distributed throughout your whole foot.

SETUP Place a mini loop band around your shins about halfway up to your knees. Then, place a long band on the ground and stand with your big toes on it, stretching the band slightly. Place feet shoulder-width apart or a little wider and turned out slightly. Extend your arms in front of you.

STEP 1 Keeping your chest proud, inhale to bend your knees as you sink your hips like you're sitting in a chair, keeping your weight over your feet. Maintain tension against the band to feel the outside of your glutes engage. Focus on pushing the band out and keeping your big toes on the band on the ground.

STEP 2 Exhale to push yourself back up controlling the tension in the band. Continue for the prescribed amount of time.

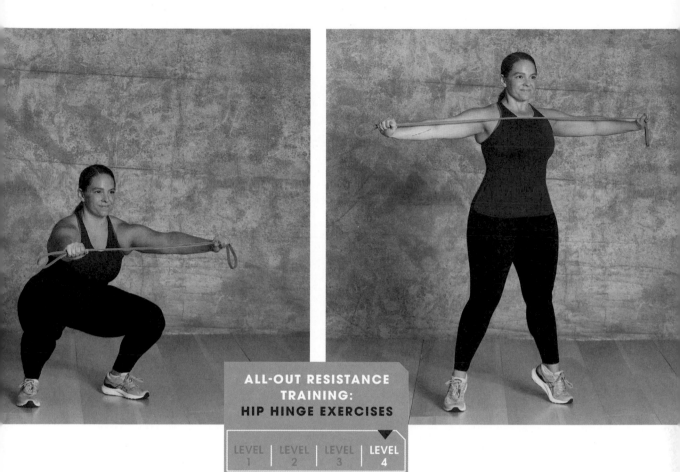

ALL-OUT RESISTANCE TRAINING: HIP HINGE EXERCISES

LEVEL 1	LEVEL 2	LEVEL 3	LEVEL 4

SQUATS TO HEEL RAISES WITH PULL-APARTS

SETUP Stand with feet shoulder-width apart or a little wider and turned out slightly. Hold the ends of a long loop in your hands, palms face down with arms stretched out in front of you.

STEP 1 Keeping your chest proud, inhale to bend your knees as you sink your hips like you're sitting in a chair, keeping your weight over your feet.

STEP 2 Exhale to push yourself back up.

STEP 3 Lift your heels off the ground.

STEP 4 Return to standing and pull the band apart.

STEP 5 Bring your arms back in front of you. Continue for the prescribed amount of time.

All Out Resistance Training

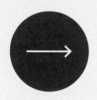

Single-Leg Exercises

Hip airplanes combine the best of a whole range of different exercises, so it's the only move you'll do for every level of your All Out single-leg series. It builds stability as you work to prevent the band from pulling your standing leg inward and it increases mobility strength as you push against the band to raise your working knee.

This exercise can be challenging to master, which is also why you won't learn any variations of it in this series. Number one rule: No pain! You should feel a really nice burn in the outer part of your glutes, but if you experience pain try lifting your leg a little lower or learning the move seated—doing the same knee-opening motion while sitting on a chair can help get you started. Your body will figure it out eventually. Trust it and trust yourself!

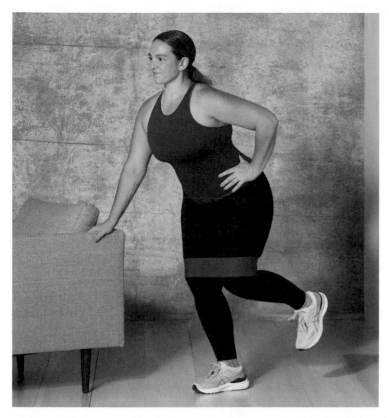

HIP AIRPLANES

SETUP Stand slightly less than arm's-length from a wall or back of a couch, right hand on the back of the couch, feet hip-width apart. Place a mini loop just above the bend of your knees.

STEP 1 Shift your head, chest, and hips over your right foot, raising your left foot until your shin is parallel to the ground. Slightly bend your right knee so you can hinge into your hips and feel a slight stretching sensation in your right glute.

STEP 2 Inhale anchoring your shoulder blades down.

STEP 3 Exhale forcefully using your glutes to explosively lift your left knee out and up. Pause for 3 to 5 seconds feeling your outer glutes.

STEP 4 Inhale to control the return to the starting position. Continue for the prescribed amount of time then repeat on the opposite side.

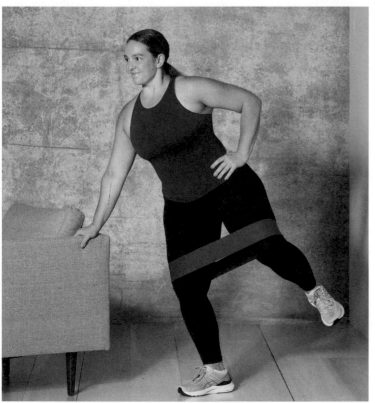

All Out Resistance Training

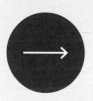

Core Exercises

Some of the most well-known core exercises—situps, crunches, bicycles—rely on a specific action to activate your abs: curling your back. However, when done lying down, this position can cause discomfort for many people. It puts a lot of strain on your neck as you fight gravity to elevate your shoulders. In this core series, you'll tap into that same curled position but without the stress and tension on your neck. Instead of curling up, you'll curl down, using the resistance from the band to challenge your abs. It's a gentler—but just as effective—way to build a strong and powerful core.

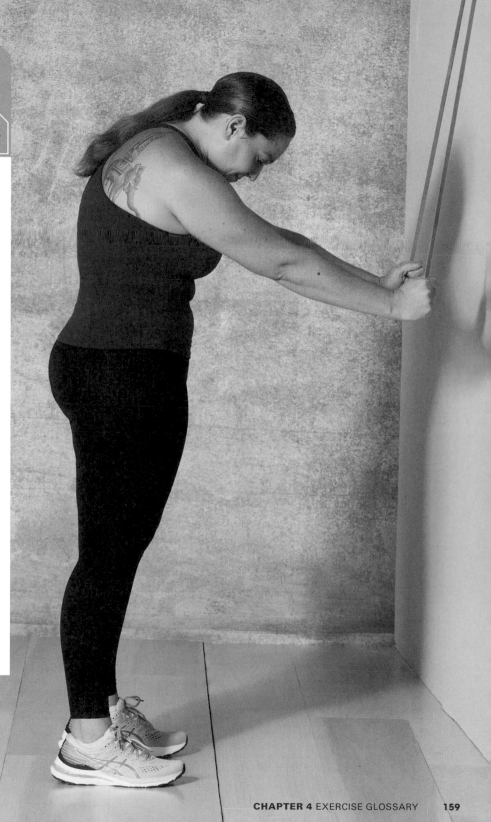

| LEVEL 1 | LEVEL 2 | LEVEL 3 | LEVEL 4 |

STANDING AB CURL PULL-DOWNS

SETUP Anchor a long loop or long band to a doorknob or bar. Grip the band in each hand, palms facing each other, arms straight out in front of you at shoulder height. You can have a slight bend in the elbows but try to keep them stiff. Stand with feet hip-width apart.

STEP 1 Inhale, pushing your ribs out.

STEP 2 Exhale, keeping your arms straight, bend forward slightly, curling your back on the way down, like you would during a crunch. Pull the band downward as you bend.

STEP 3 Return to the starting position. Continue for the prescribed amount of time.

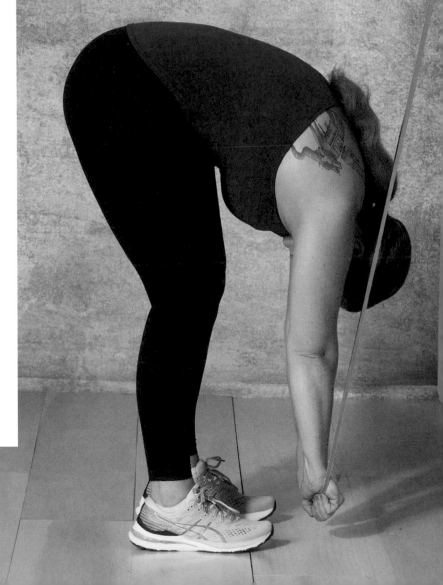

LEVEL 1	LEVEL 2	LEVEL 3	LEVEL 4

STANDING AB CURL PUSH-DOWNS

SETUP Anchor either a long loop or an open band to a doorknob or a bar. Grip the band in each hand, palms down, arms out in front of you at shoulder height. You can have a slight bend in the elbows but try to keep them stiff. Stand with feet hip-width apart.

STEP 1 Inhale, standing tall with a slight bend in your knees, then slowly exhale, pushing the band toward your feet and bending forward as you go, trying to roll down the spine one vertebrae at a time.

STEP 2 Inhale again at the bottom, then exhale to roll back up the spine continuing to push the band toward the floor. Continue for the prescribed amount of time.

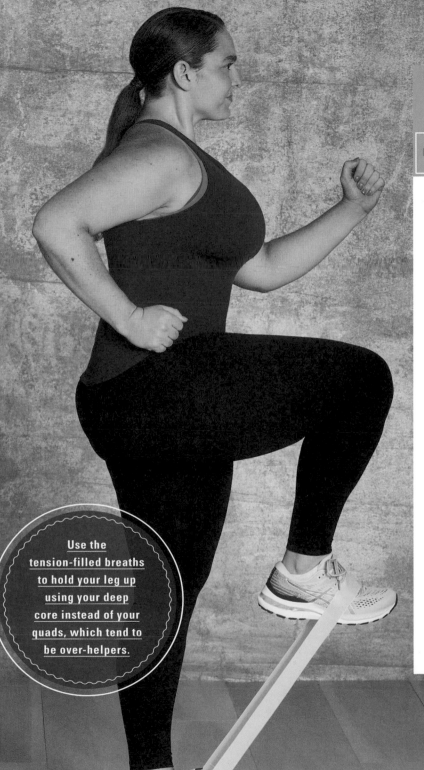

ISOMETRIC BANDED STANDING MARCHING

SETUP Stand with feet shoulder-width apart. Place a mini loop around the arches of your feet.

STEP 1 Inhale to shift your head, chest, and hips over your left foot.

STEP 2 Exhale to slowly lift your right knee up, aiming to raise it parallel to the ground by the end of your exhale. Using short, tension-filled breaths, aim to hold this position for the prescribed amount of time.

STEP 3 Return to the starting position. Repeat on the opposite side.

> Use the tension-filled breaths to hold your leg up using your deep core instead of your quads, which tend to be over-helpers.

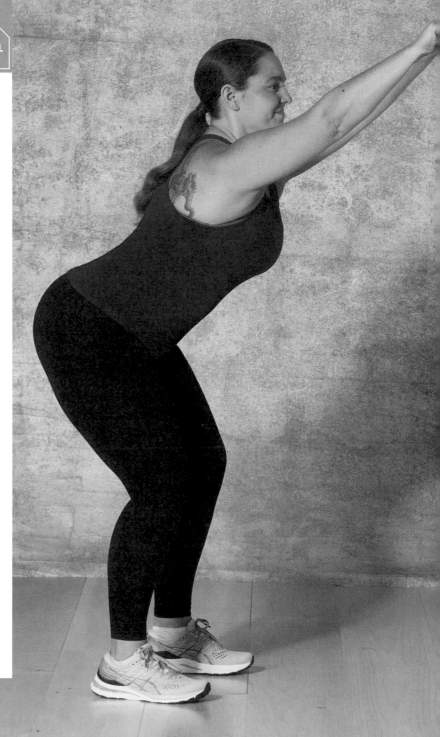

ISOMETRIC BENT-OVER LAT PULL-DOWNS

SETUP Anchor either a long loop or an open band to a doorknob or a bar. Grip the band in each hand, palms face out, arms out in front of you at shoulder height. You can have a slight bend in the elbows but try to keep them stiff.

STEP 1 Walk your feet back and slightly wider—like your squat stance—and hinge your hips behind you until you find your arms create one long line from your shoulder to where your band is anchored.

STEP 2 Inhale, anchoring your shoulder blades toward your hips. Exhale, pull your elbows into your sides and hands into your upper arms.

STEP 3 Using a short tension-filled breath, hold this position for the prescribed amount of time, trying to squeeze your shoulder blades low and together.

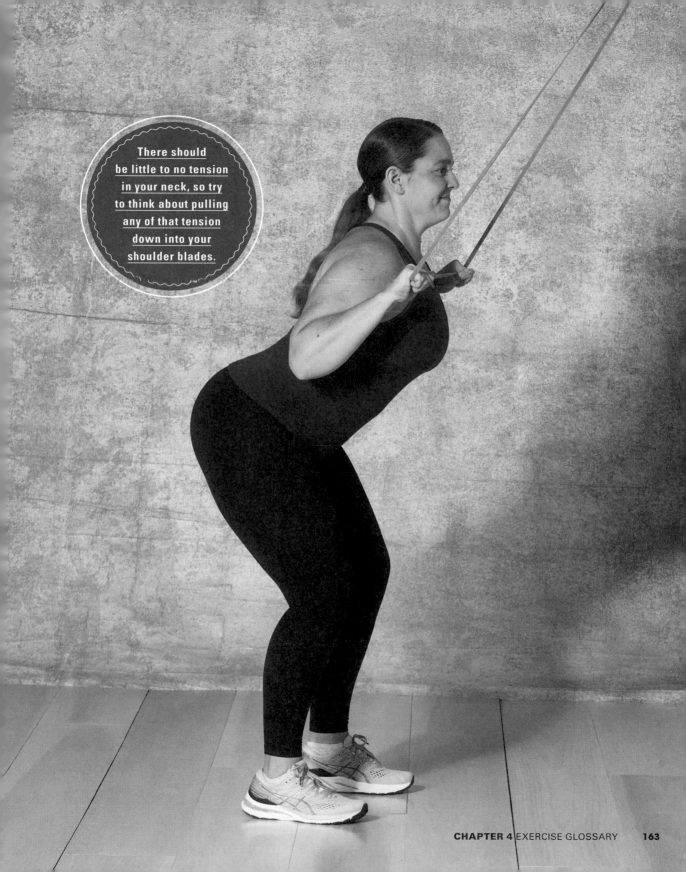

There should be little to no tension in your neck, so try to think about pulling any of that tension down into your shoulder blades.

Cardio+ Exercises

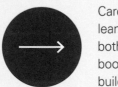

Cardio and resistance training are essential to getting lean and toned and this series gives you the best of both worlds. You'll get your whole body moving (and boost your heart rate!) while also sneaking in muscle-building moves, like lunges and squats. Think of it as your supercharged workout! If you're struggling to maintain your form, drop the band and focus on mastering the movement before adding in more resistance. I've left out any breathing cues here—it's hard enough completing these move as is, so breathe however comes naturally. However, if you need a little extra oomph to get through this series, try forcefully exhaling at the hardest part of the exercise. This'll help you engage your core and power through. Experiment with deep breathing and short, tension-filled breaths until you find what works for you.

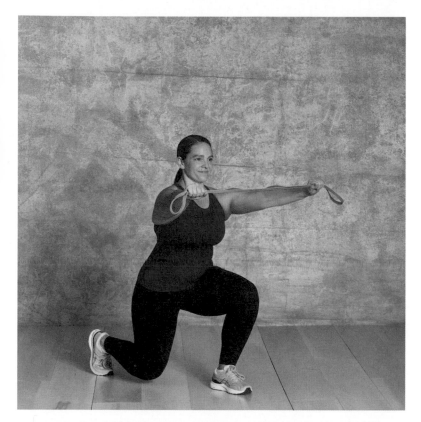

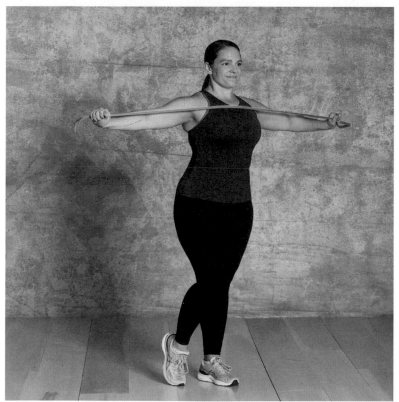

ALTERNATING REVERSE LUNGES WITH PULL-APARTS

SETUP Stand with feet hip-width and hold a long loop in both hands, arms extended in front of you at shoulder height, palms facing down.

STEP 1 Step your right foot straight back behind you, planting the ball of your foot and dropping your right knee toward the floor, sitting straight down into both feet.

STEP 2 Push yourself up, planting the ball of your right foot next to your left foot.

STEP 3 Anchor your shoulder blades and pull the band apart, squeezing your shoulder blades together behind you.

STEP 4 Bring your arms back in front of you. Repeat on the opposite side. Continue alternating sides for the prescribed amount of time.

MOUNTAIN CLIMBERS

SETUP Place a mini loop band around the arches of your feet, hip-width apart. Place your hands on the back of a couch or wall and walk your feet away until you're in one long line leaning toward your hands.

STEP 1 Draw your right knee in toward your ribs, keeping your foot flexed to keep the band in place.

STEP 2 In one smooth, controlled motion switch knees.

STEP 3 Continue alternating sides for the prescribed amount of time.

If you're struggling to alternate feet quickly, hold the raised knee for 1 to 3 seconds then plant both feet on the ground before repeating on the other side.

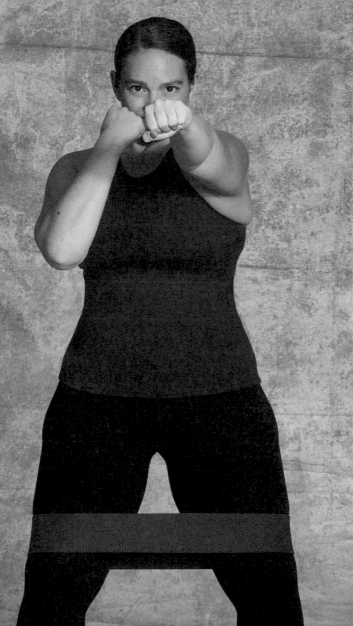

BOXING JABS

SETUP Place a mini loop around your legs, just above the bend in your knees. Stand with feet slightly wider than shoulder-width, pulling tension outward in the band. Make fists or hold small weights or soup cans in each hand In front of you at chin level.

STEP 1 Maintain tension in the band as you jab your left fist out in front and pull it back with control as quickly as possible.

STEP 2 Alternate your hands with quick jabs thinking about "throwing" from your shoulder blades and maintaining tension in the band throughout the prescribed amount of time.

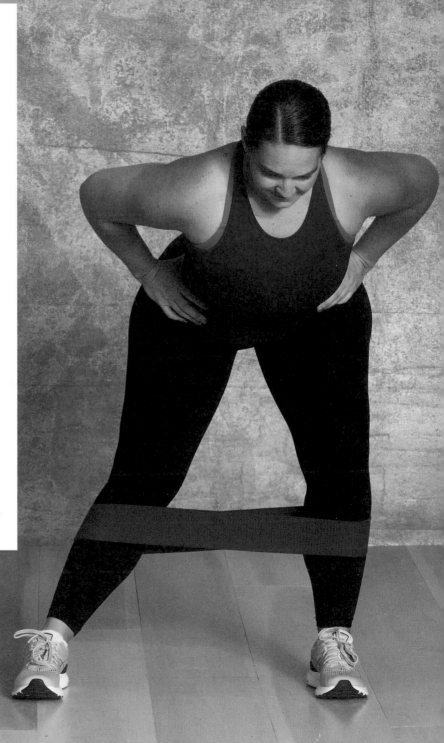

LATERAL LUNGES

SETUP Place a mini loop band around your legs just below the knee. Stand tall with feet hip-width apart, hands can hang by your sides or rest on your hips.

STEP 1 Take a wide step with the left foot to the side pushing the band out to prevent the band from pulling the knee in. As you step to the side, sit your hips back and reach your proud chest forward to stay square as you bend the left knee and shift your three major weights (head, chest, hips) over your left foot.

STEP 2 Push through the left foot to return back to the starting position, control bringing the right leg back in. Continue for the prescribed amount of time then repeat on the opposite side.

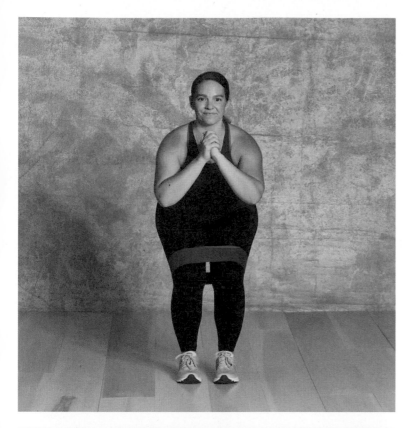

POP SQUATS

SETUP Place a mini loop band around your legs just above the knees and stand tall, feet hip-width apart. Arms can move naturally or you can clasp your hands at your chest.

STEP 1 Sit halfway into your squat and aim to stay this low throughout the entire prescribed time.

STEP 2 Push against the band to "pop" or shoot your feet into a wider stance and to hop them back to the narrow starting stance.

STEP 3 Continue to hop out and back in for the prescribed amount of time.

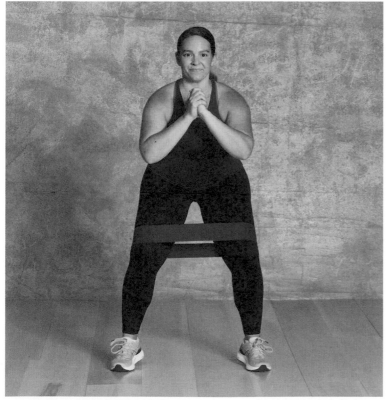

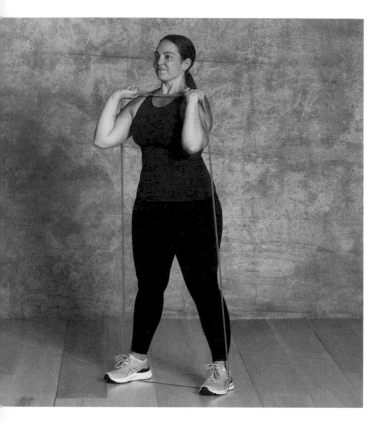
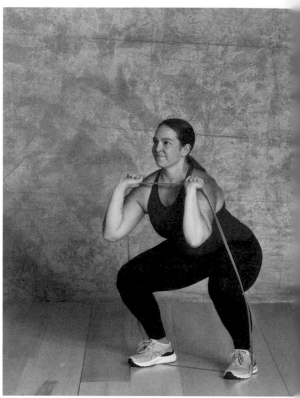

THRUSTERS

SETUP Stand with feet shoulder-width apart, a long loop band taut under both feet and held in each hand at shoulder height, palms facing up, elbows pointing forward.

STEP 1 Sit into your squat, reaching your elbows forward.

STEP 2 Stand back up and use the momentum to help you push the band overhead.

STEP 3 Bend the elbows to bring the band back to shoulder height to sit back into your squat. Continue for the prescribed amount of time.

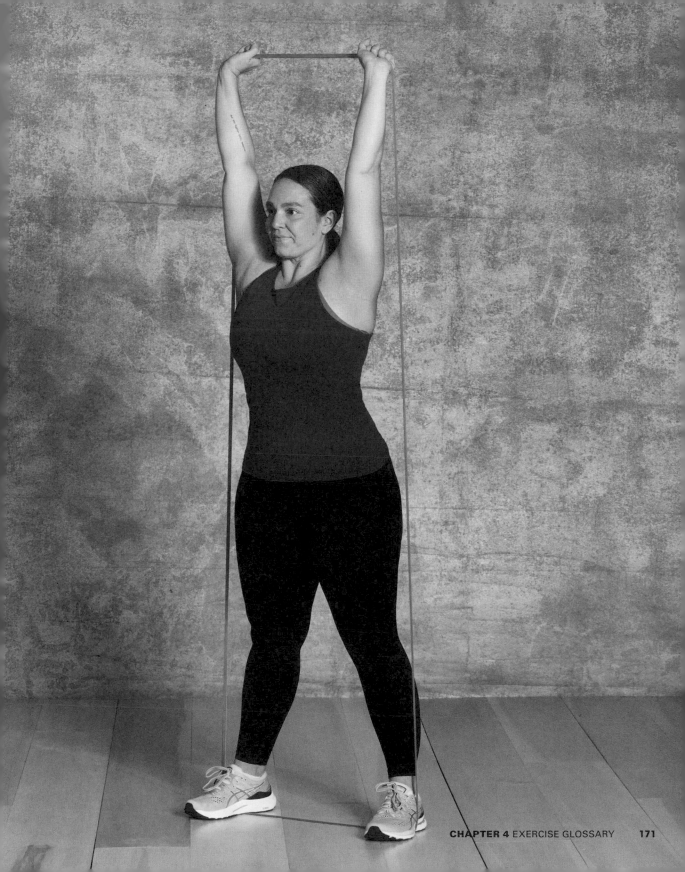

Total-Body Reset Exercises

These exercises are all about doing what feels good for you. Feel free to start the triangle lunge series with a chair under your butt for the most support and stability. On days when you have more time and want to get deeper, try to find the push and pull of the stretch. In your triangle lunges you can do this by pushing into your feet to straighten your legs as much as possible, then pulling your hips down and wide to sit into the deep lunge.

In the second step of the triangle lunge series, aim to keep your heels down, which might mean you need to come up out of the depth a bit. Here the push and pull happens simultaneously for the external rotators of the hips, so push into the big toe to squeeze your glute and try to pull the bent knee as much as you can. Shift over to the other side however you like. You can try and challenge your hip mobility by seeing how low you can shift over.

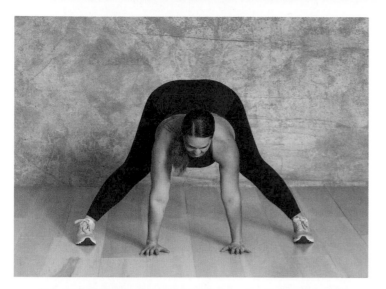

TRIANGLE LUNGE SERIES

SETUP Stand with your feet as wide as you like and bend over, placing your hands on the ground, a couch, or the wall for support.

STEP 1 Turn your right leg in while bending and turning your left leg out, placing your hands to the right of your left foot. Your hips, knees, and feet should all be pointing the same direction. Hold for at least 40 seconds.

STEP 2 Gently rotate your hips to the right until your right knee faces up, bringing your upper body with you, hands in front of you. Keep your left knee over your middle toes. Hold for at least 40 seconds.

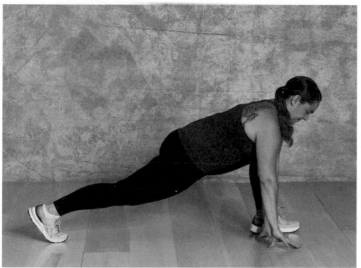

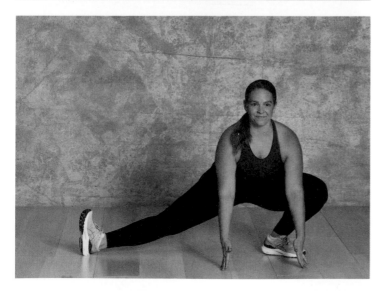

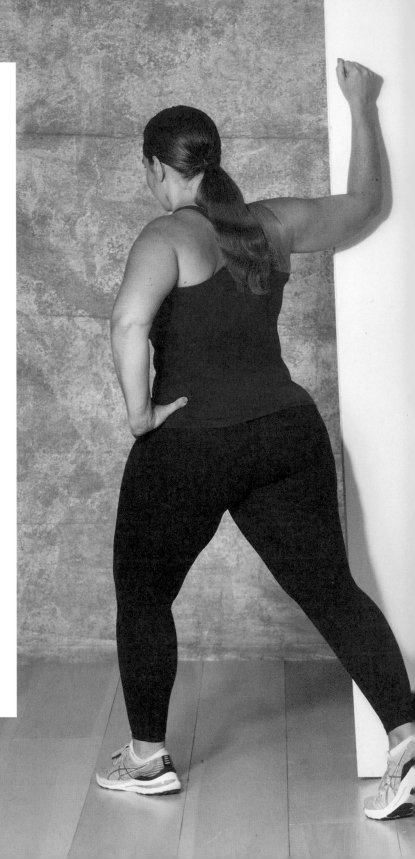

DOORWAY UPPER-BODY STRETCH

SETUP Find a doorway or pillar and stand just off to the side with your elbow against the doorway, shoulder height, fist stacked at a 90-degree bend on top of the elbow.

STEP 1 Anchor the shoulders just like with our upper body lifts, gently walk a few steps forward through the doorway to stretch along the front of your body and arm.

STEP 2 From here, anchor the shoulder and try to pull your fist away from the doorway, keeping your elbow from moving. Hold the farthest range you can get for 3 to 5 seconds before returning to the start.

STEP 3 Once you've done both sides, stand slightly to the side of the doorway. Grab the doorway with both hands, the outside hand being on top.

STEP 4 Lean your weight into your hips, away from the doorway, creating a banana or boat shape with your whole body.

STEP 5 Inhale and exhale into your side and the side of your back rib cage to find the push and pull.

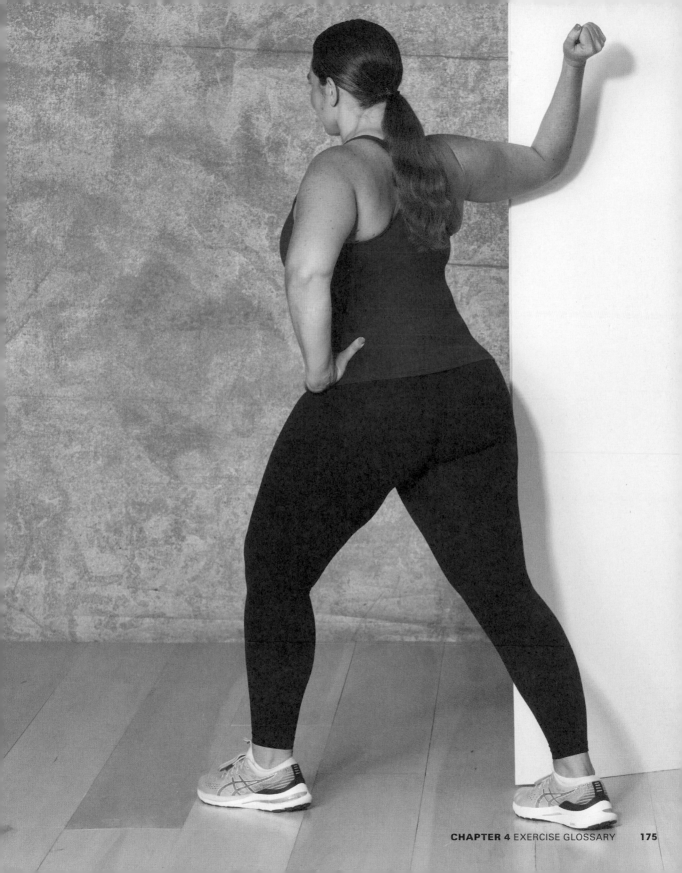

NOTES

Resources

BOOKS

18 Minutes by Peter Bregman
Strong Women Lift Each Other Up by Molly Galbraith
GirlsGoneStrong Pre/Post Natal Certification Guidebook
10,000 Hours by Malcolm Gladwell
Rebuilding Milo by Aaron Horschig and Kevin Sonthana
Lifting Heavy Things by Laura Khoudari
When the Body Says No by Gabor Maté

INSTAGRAM ACCOUNTS

@disabledgirlswholift
@handi_capable_fitness
@harlemkettlebellclub
@kympossible_fitness
@laurenleavellfitness
@squatuniversity
@syattfitness
@tiffanyima

PODCASTS

Maintenance Phase

WEB PAGES

"Functional Movement Screens/Assessment"
functionalmovement.com/store/35/fms_level_1_online_course

"Functional Anatomy Courses"
brookbushinstitute.com/courses

"Mobility Fundamentals"
rehab-u.com/courses/mobility-fundamentals/

"The Binge and the Brain"
dana.org/article/the-binge-and-the-brain/

"Girls Gone Strong"
girlsgonestrong.com/blog/category/free-courses/

VIDEOS

Sensory Minis- Proprioception
youtube.com/watch?v=Oquc160D1dw

PHOTO CREDITS

Cover photography by
Philip Friedman

Interior photography by
Philip Friedman: 6, 8, 18, 28, 31,
38, 40, 42, 44, 46, 48, 49, 50, 52,
54, 56-58, 60-62, 64-66, 68-175;
Getty Images: 1shot Production/
E+: 30; Alexandr Screaghin/iStock:
25; Anastassiya Bezhekeneva/
Moment: 41; blackCAT/E+: 21;
Dean Mitchell/E+: 22; FatCamera/
E+: 43; Gpointstudio/Image Source:
24; jacoblund/iStock: 67; Malorny/
Moment: 33; mixetto/E+: 55;
mladenbalinovac/E+: 17; Nikola
Ilic/E+: 14; Patrik Giardino/Stone:
12; Prostock-Studio/iStock: 32;
Scvos/iStock: 33; Scvos/iStock: 33;
SDI Productions/E+: 63; The Good
Brigade/DigitalVision: 180; The Noun
Project: 20; urbazon/E+: 59; Victor
Tkachev/iStock: 33; Westend61:
10, 47, 51; Zorica Nastasic/E+: 39

This book is intended as a reference volume only, not as a medical manual. The information given here is designed to help you make informed decisions about your health. It is not intended as a substitute for any treatment that may have been prescribed by your doctor. If you suspect that you have a medical problem, we urge you to seek competent medical help.

Mention of specific companies, organizations, or authorities in this book does not imply endorsement by the author or publisher, nor does mention of specific companies, organizations, or authorities imply that they endorse this book, its author, or the publisher.

Prevention is a registered trademark of Hearst Magazines, Inc.

Book design by Michael Wilson

Library of Congress Cataloging-in-Publication Data is on file with the publisher.

ISBN 978-1-955710-29-9

Printed in China

2 4 6 8 10 9 7 5 3 1 hardcover

HEARST